Towards Evidence-based Suicide Prevention Programmes

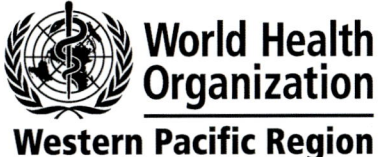

WHO Library Cataloguing in Publication Data

Towards evidence-based suicide prevention programmes.

1. Suicide - prevention and control.

ISBN 978 92 9061 462 3   (NLM Classification: W822)

© World Health Organization 2010

All rights reserved. Publications of the World Health Organization can be obtained from WHO Press, World Health Organization, 20 Avenue Appia, 1211 Geneva 27, Switzerland (tel.: +41 22 791 3264; fax: +41 22 791 4857; e-mail: bookorders@who.int). Requests for permission to reproduce or translate WHO publications – whether for sale or for noncommercial distribution – should be addressed to WHO Press, at the above address (fax: +41 22 791 4806; e-mail: permissions@who.int).   For WHO Western Pacific Regional Publications, request for permission to reproduce should be addressed to the Publications Office, World Health Organization, Regional Office for the Western Pacific, P.O. Box 2932, 1000, Manila, Philippines, Fax. No. (632) 521-1036, email: publications@wpro.who.int

The designations employed and the presentation of the material in this publication do not imply the expression of any opinion whatsoever on the part of the World Health Organization concerning the legal status of any country, territory, city or area or of its authorities, or concerning the delimitation of its frontiers or boundaries. Dotted lines on maps represent approximate border lines for which there may not yet be full agreement.

The mention of specific companies or of certain manufacturers' products does not imply that they are endorsed or recommended by the World Health Organization in preference to others of a similar nature that are not mentioned. Errors and omissions excepted, the names of proprietary products are distinguished by initial capital letters.

All reasonable precautions have been taken by the World Health Organization to verify the information contained in this publication. However, the published material is being distributed without warranty of any kind, either expressed or implied. The responsibility for the interpretation and use of the material lies with the reader. In no event shall the World Health Organization be liable for damages arising from its use.

Table of Contents

Preface v

Acknowledgements viii

Chapter 1: Introduction 1

    The public health approach 3

        The public health approach processes 5

        Illustration of public health approach in suicide prevention 7

        The public health approach in practice 8

Chapter 2: Formulation and evaluation of suicide prevention programmes 9

    Need for effective suicide prevention programmes 9

    Key elements in formulating suicide prevention strategies 10

        Comprehensiveness 10

        Empirical evidence 10

        Measurable outcomes 10

        Subject to change 10

        Sustainability 11

    Criteria for effective interventions 11

        Empirically established conceptual framework 11

        Clear identification of target individuals 11

        Carefully planned intervention/preventative measures 11

        Systematic evaluation 12

    Measurable outcome indicators for interventions 12

        Major outcomes for interventions 12

  Associated outcomes for interventions..13

 Examples of evidence-based suicide prevention programmes 15

  Worldwide 16

  Western Pacific Region...27

Chapter 3: A snapshot of suicide prevention interventions in the
Western Pacific Region 37

Chapter 4: Priority...51

 Surveillance and monitoring 52

 Epidemiologic research 52

 Evidence-based prevention and intervention programmes..................................52

  Universal level..53

  Selective level...53

  Indicated level 54

 Evaluation...54

References...56

Preface

Suicide is a global challenge. It poses a serious public health problem worldwide. It has accounted for nearly 1 million deaths and an estimated 10 million attempted suicides each year. It is estimated that approximately 32% of all suicide deaths have occurred in the Western Pacific Region (Hendin *et al.* 2008, Yip 2008), which is disproportionately found in this area consisting of 37 countries and areas with a total of 1.78 billion people or about 29% of the world's population. It is estimated that, in this Region, the suicide rate is calculated to be about 19.3 per 100,000 (De Leo, Milner and Wang 2009). Suicide rates in some countries/areas like Japan, the Republic of Korea and Taiwan, China have had significant increases recently and remained at historically high levels. Suicide is the leading cause of death among young people in this Region and has caused significant economic losses to society. The full impact of the world's current economic crisis has yet to be realized, but it's certain to have an effect on mental health and suicide. It is unfortunate as well that suicide prevention resources are limited and underdeveloped, especially in developing countries, which have the largest need for resources and help.

This monograph attempts to set out the basic framework for suicide prevention strategies. It provides details in formulating and evaluating suicide prevention programmes. The public health approaches suggested offer a multilayer intervention model, which has been adopted by a number of developed countries for setting up national prevention strategies. Nevertheless, we want to stress that there is no single solution in dealing with suicide in a heterogeneous environment: one size simply doesn't fit all. Also, all suicide prevention programmes need to be evaluated. And where we do not have the necessary evidence, we must simultaneously implement novel approaches and rigorously evaluate them. Anything less is undesirable. The importance of evaluation is even more critical in Asia, partly due to culture and limited resources.

We have included the details of some well-established suicide prevention programmes worldwide and in the Western Pacific Region. They have been shown effective in reducing the number of suicides and/or its associated outcome indicators. We hope that by publishing this monograph more cultural-specific programmes on suicide prevention can be developed in the Region. The more we know, the more we can learn from one another about effective suicide prevention strategies. The need for suicide prevention is increasing, especially in the populous countries in the Region. The applicability of the public health approaches for suicide prevention in developing countries has yet to be established due to the diverse economic and sociocultural backgrounds.

There are significant differences in resource availability in implementing suicide prevention programmes among countries in the Region. We highlight important features of some evidence-based programmes. Recognizing the many factors that put people at risk of suicide and protecting them against those factors, we believe that only strategies from multiple levels and disciplines can help in reducing suicides substantially. Effective actions should be evidence-based and multilayered. The effectiveness of prevention programmes should also be evaluated by measurable outcomes. In addition, programmes should be adaptive and open for improvement based on the evaluation results.

This monograph outlines fundamental principles, many of which have been ignored in the past, to develop community suicide prevention programmes. We advocate the formulation of a task force that will lead the implementation of an operational plan and develop schedules for a coordinated community-based suicide prevention strategies. It is not a static process but rather a continuous and evolving strategy, which advocates sustainable development on suicide prevention based on the best research knowledge available and the cooperation of all stakeholders in the community. Any nationwide suicide prevention programme ideally should be supported by government so that it works more effectively among all the stakeholders in the community. The task force should be financially sustainable. Moreover, partnership and cooperation will be emphasized, building upon many activities within the community that have already contributed to suicide prevention. Suicide prevention is multidimensional, whether we are speaking of the need to tailor diverse solutions for different cultures or develop distinctive approaches for various segments of the population within a country. In other words, "one size doesn't fit all". Each of us must develop culturally attuned, locally relevant and evidence-based suicide prevention programmes.

Preface

We have seen some significant progress in understanding suicide and its prevention in Hong Kong (China) over the past 10 years. We wish to share some of our research experiences (both successful and unsuccessful) into coordinated strategies. This monograph aims to extend current knowledge and promote ongoing discourse within the community and in the Region. The guidance in this document needs to be continuously updated and modified, and we must remain open and responsive in light of new discussions and evidence. We cannot emphasize any more that "suicide is everyone's business." It is only when individuals representing every facet of our communities come together and work together to confront this serious problem can the tragedies and sufferings of affected families and friends be reduced. Minimizing the number of suicides has always been a challenge. However, by using available resources effectively while identifying new resources, we certainly can make a difference.

Acknowledgements

The Western Pacific region of the WHO gratefully acknowledges the authors who wrote this monograph: Professor Paul S.F. Yip & Ms Yik-wa Law, both affiliated with Centre for Suicide Research & Prevention, University of Hong Kong.

Paul Yip is the Director of the Centre for Suicide Research and Prevention (CSRP) and a professor of the Department of Social Work & Social Administration, the University of Hong Kong (HKU). He is also the Vice-President of the International Association for Suicide Prevention. Y.W. Law is a social worker and a Ph.D. Candidate (HKU) who has been actively involved in developing suicide prevention programmes. She is also a core team member of CSRP, HKU and is appointed as a Professional Member of the China National Suicide Prevention and Crisis Intervention Association.

Special thanks are given to Dr King-wa Fu, Journalism and Media Studies Centre and Dr Paul W.C. Wong, Centre for Suicide Research & Prevention, the University of Hong Kong for their intellectual inputs, and Mr Philip Jean-Richard Dit Bressel and Miss Claudine L. Ying for their research support in preparing this monograph.

Chapter 1: Introduction

Suicide is a serious global public health problem, with nearly 1 million individuals committing suicide each year (World Health Organization 2010a). The burden of suicide is also unevenly distributed. For example, more than 60% of these suicides occur in Asia (Beautrais 2006, Yip 2008). The People's Republic of China, with its large population, is estimated to account for about 25% of total suicide deaths globally (Yip, Liu, and Law 2008). There is diversity in cultural and socioeconomic development, and thus many countries in Asia have considerable differences in suicide patterns. For example, suicide rates in this Region vary from below 5 per 100 000 like in the Philippines (2.1 per 100 000) to above 20 per 100 000 in Japan (24.4), and the Republic of Korea (21.9) (World Health Organization 2010b). It is estimated that, in the Region, the suicide rates are calculated to be about 19.3 per 100 000, which is 30% higher than the global suicide rates (De Leo, Milner and Wang 2009). Due to rapid transitions of the social and economic structures experienced by many countries in the Region, and given the limited resources of mental health services, suicide rates are predicted to worsen in the next two decades.

Considerable differences in suicide rates are often found within groups in the same country, such as those in the rural and urban areas, males and females, the young and the elderly, etc. Some of these prevalent distributions contrast with the distributions in well-researched Western countries. Consequently, over-reliance on Western research for suicide prevention in the Western Pacific Region should be avoided. For instance, the People's Republic of China has a unique gender suicide ratio, with more female suicides than males, and higher rural than urban suicide rates, which are the opposite in Western countries (Phillips, Li and Zhang 2002, Phillips, Liu and Zhang 1999, Yip, Callanan and Yuen 2000). These patterns found in the People's Republic of China cannot be generalized to neighbouring areas. Even Hong Kong (China), a former British colony, has different epidemiological data. Each country has a unique epidemiological profile and must be studied individually and thoroughly to understand its suicide patterns. Along with suicide distributions, there are also unique patterns to suicide methods. Hanging and jumping from high places are common, like in Western countries. However, some Asia-specific methods, such as poisoning by pesticides, or carbon monoxide poisoning through charcoal burning in confined spaces, are unique and present unique challenges for suicide prevention efforts in the Region. Also, suicide is a contagious, creating a copycat effect due to the sensational reporting by the media that is particularly serious in Asia (Chen *et al.* 2010, Fu and Yip 2008). Suicide methods can then be "learnt" by other countries through media reporting (Chan *et al.* 2005 Yip and Lee 2007).

For any suicide prevention research programme, the most important piece of information is the fundamental measure of the suicide rates (number of suicide per 100 000). Unfortunately, the definition of suicide is unclear in some geographic areas. We cannot simply take it for granted that there is an accurate description of the suicide phenomenon based on the existing data. It is still a major challenge for the epidemiologist, as well as suicide prevention scientist in this area. It is not likely that a resolution will be found in a short period of time. Both the case definition and the procedure correcting for the error inherent in suicide data vary widely, highlighting the need to establish a measurement standard (Claassen *et al.* 2009).

An important consideration is how suicide statistics are obtained. This also varies between countries, with the most reliable suicide data found in countries that have an established, validated coronial system for establishing the cause of death for each individual (e.g. Japan, Australia, New Zealand, Hong Kong (China), Singapore, the Republic of Korea, and Malaysia). Some countries rely on estimates extrapolated from population sampling, i.e. the People's Republic of China, which does not require the cause of death to be recorded outside of hospitals; or Viet Nam, providing relatively unreliable data to work with (Hendin *et al.* 2008). The variation in recording cause of death information across different countries in the Region may hinder research into suicide and its prevention (De Leo 2002).

Other confounding variables are the cultural and religious elements which affect the reporting of suicide. For instance, suicide is prohibited by the dominant religions in the Region (e.g. Islam, Buddhism, Hinduism, and Christianity), and is even illegal in some countries, i.e. Malaysia, possibly because of historical and religious reasons, or because it reflects negatively on society. Data collection methods and socioeconomic/cultural factors leave much room for intentional and unintentional misclassification and underreporting of suicide. It is widely agreed by experts that suicide is significantly underreported in countries with poor death classification systems and social intolerances for suicide (Beautrais 2006, Hendin *et al.* 2008, Vijayakumar *et al.* 2005b, Yip 2008, Yip *et al.* 2005). This points to an even more alarming issue than initial data suggest.

The burden of suicide death is unevenly distributed. Despite the fact that the majority of suicides occur in Asia, 90% of all worldwide suicide research is spent on 10% of the suicide population which resides in other parts of the world, i.e. the United States of America and Western Europe. Even with a strong rationale to encourage evidence-based interventions and context-specific research in the Region, lack of resources and competing priorities have left suicide prevention fragmented. Though it is evident that the problem of suicide has significant social, economic and health impact in different societies, Western Pacific countries have done relatively little to combat the epidemic. There is, however, in Taiwan, China, the Republic of Korea, and some cities in the southern regions of the People's Republic of China, such as Shenzhen, and Hong Kong (China) an encouraging trend of greater acknowledgement by the government, or local community leaders, and professional groups. This is a vital step towards implementing effective and comprehensive suicide prevention strategies.

The public health approach

In the past few decades, there were huge advances in the theory and practice of public health strategies for the prevention and intervention in behaviour-related mortality and morbidity. Traditionally, suicide has been viewed as a mental health issue addressed primarily through clinical interventions, especially in the treatment of depression (Mercy and Rosenberg 2000). However, it has been found that the majority of people who committed suicide did not receive psychiatric services prior to death (Andersen *et al.* 2000, Appleby *et al.* 1999, Cavanagh *et al.* 2003, Lee *et al.* 2008). People who committed suicide were found almost three times as likely to have been unable to get the needed medical care compared to those who died by other causes of death (Miller and Druss 2001). In other words, even individual patients can benefit from effective intervention. An estimated 25% to 50% of the suicide population can be reached, which is far from satisfactory.

Based on rigorous calculations (Lewis, Hawton and Jones 1997), it has been shown that high-risk clinical strategies only have a modest effect on a population's suicide rates, even if effective interventions are developed. The United Kingdom government's target for suicide reduction would more likely be achieved using population-based strategies aimed at actively reducing risks among the whole population. Furthermore, many studies point out that suicide could be an interplay of a wide array of factors, including biological or genetic, sociocultural, psychological, and behavioural factors (Hawton and van Heeringen 2009). It is thus imperative that in addition to improving effectiveness of clinical interventions, multiple avenues should be utilized to prevent suicide deaths, particularly in populous countries, such as those in the Western Pacific Region. In the Region, mental health services can hardly meet the huge demand of populations due to limited resources and stigmatization towards mental health service in the community.

The public health approach focuses on identifying the patterns of suicide and suicidal behaviours of a group or population. It aims at changing the environment to protect people against diseases and changing the behaviours that put people at risk of getting diseases. The public health approach is not limited to epidemic diseases but can also be applied to solving the suicide problem. Suicide was tackled as a public health problem since the early 1980s in the United States of America by the Centre for Health Promotion and Education (CHPE) under the Centers for Disease Control and Prevention (CDC). It did so by installing a surveillance system, which was developed to estimate the occurrence of suicide across the nation (Mercy and Rosenberg 2000). Since then, there has been concerted effort to advocate a public health approach to the suicide problem, which focuses on identifying suicide patterns and suicidal behaviour in a group or population (Cantor and Baume 1999, Hammond 2001, Hoven *et al.* 2009, Knox, Conwell and Caine 2004, Lewis, Hawton and Jones 1997, Mercy and Rosenberg 2000, Potter, Powell and Kachur 1995, Potter, Rosenberg and Hammond 1998, Yip 2005).

Based on this concept, many countries are developing national strategies, which are comprehensive and organized approaches to marshalling preventive efforts. Effective evaluation is an essential component. For example, legislation restricting pack sizes of paracetamol and salicylates in the United Kingdom serves as a good example of using the public health approach to effectively deal with the suicide problem (Hawton *et al.* 2001) (see Chapter 2).

The public health approach processes

The public health approach consists of the four processes (Figure 1).

Figure 1: Public health approach

(Mercy and Rosenberg 2000, Potter, Powell, and Kachur 1995, Potter, Rosenberg, and Hammond 1998, US Department of Health and Human Services 2001)

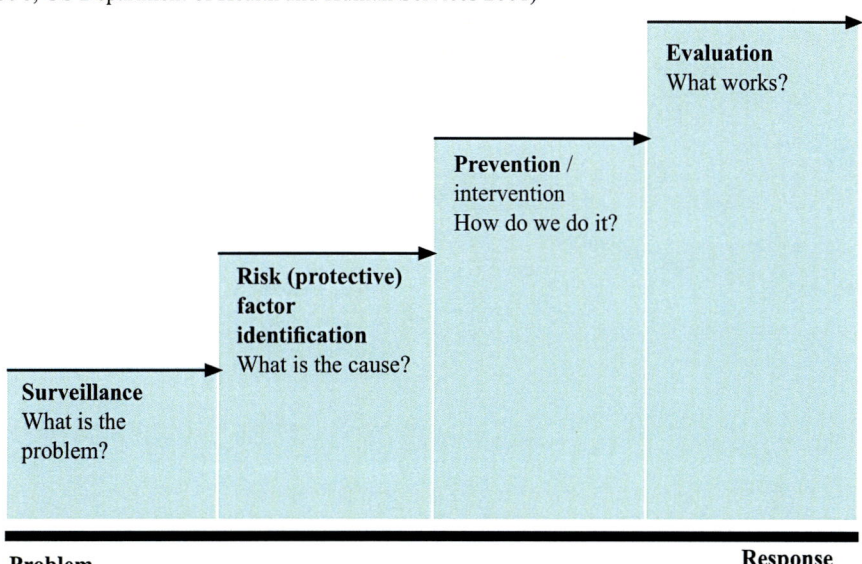

Here we illustrate in detail how the public health approach can be applied to suicide prevention:

1. **Surveillance:** It identifies suicide patterns and the different suicide rates according to age, geographical location, etc. It may also include the information on the characteristics of individuals who die by suicide. This helps to identify and define the problem.
2. **Risk (protective) factor identification:** It identifies the chain of causes leading to suicide. It includes both risk factors, which may be thought of as leading to or being associated with suicide, and protective factors, which may reduce the likelihood of such incidents, and the interaction between these factors.
3. **Prevention/intervention:** Suicide prevention efforts have been classified into three levels: universal, selective and indicated (US Department of Health and Human Services 2001) (see Table 1):

Table 1: Universal, selective, and indicated preventive interventions

Level	Definition	Examples
Universal	Affects everyone in a defined population regardless of the risk of suicide	Public education programmes about the dangers of substance abuse; public awareness of depression; limiting access to pesticide; building barriers on hotspots of suicide by jumping; and promoting responsible media reporting on suicide stories
Selective	Targets subgroups at particular suicide risk; there are a number of risk factors found related to suicide, such as mental illnesses, substance abuse, financial debts, unemployment, chronic pain for the elderly, study stress, and access to suicide means	Programmes for women in rural areas; people who are unemployed and with financial debts; young people with depressive symptoms or substance abuse problems; elderly with chronic physical illness and/or living alone; school kids with a high level of study stress; or victims of physical or sexual abuse; gatekeepers training for police, teachers, general practitioners, and community stakeholders who may identify and provide early intervention to people with possible suicide risks during their daily work
Indicated	For specific individuals who, on examination, have a risk factor or condition that puts them at very high risk, e.g. recent suicidal attempts	Crisis management or follow-up care programmes for patients with recent suicidal attempts or deliberate self-harm behaviours who have been admitted and discharged; and close monitoring measures on patients with prior suicide attempts

Altogether, these measures form a spectrum of health care interventions (Dorwart and Ostacher 1998). Experiences in Western countries suggest that more comprehensive programmes that consist of a broad mix of intervention strategies are believed to have a greater likelihood of reducing suicide rates (US Department of Health and Human Services 2001). Many of the suicide prevention works worldwide have adopted three levels of intervention. Chapter 1 provides a summary of works made according to these levels.

4. **Evaluation:** Most interventions aim to prevent suicide, but lack effectiveness in evaluation. Effectiveness is another multifaceted aspect in suicide prevention. What makes a programme effective depends on the measures and objectives of the project. This will be discussed further in Chapter 2.

An "evidence-based" approach is vital and it allows us to determine which intervention or programme is best fit for the current situation, and which is most cost-effective.

Illustration of public health approach in suicide prevention

A concept behind the public health approach is that its effect would be found throughout the whole population. To illustrate how the public health approach aims to reduce the number of suicides, a simple diagram can be used (Yip 2005). If the mental health of a population could be drawn as a normally distributed curve with the x-axis representing suicide risk and the y-axis representing the number of people, a universal programme would in theory shift the whole curve to the left (see Figure 2). This would reduce the number of individuals found in the high-risk bracket (relative to the size of the shift) while making the whole population less susceptible to suicide. Also, "a large number of people at a small risk may give rise to more cases of disease than the small numbers who are at high risk" (Rose 1992). A reduction in general risk would reduce suicide cases more than interventions that only target high-risk individuals.

Figure 2: This shows the effect of a shift in the mean suicidal risk of a population.

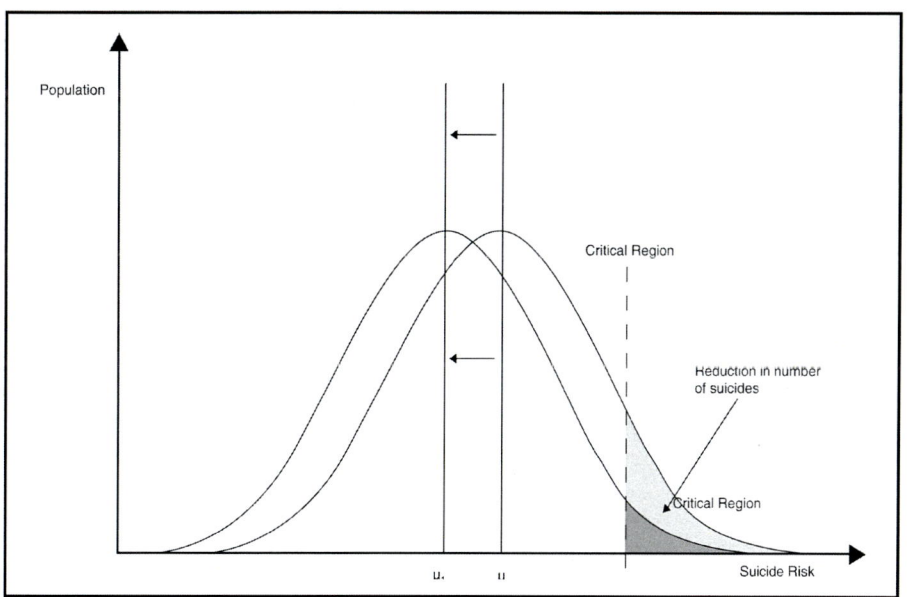

Note: μ, original population mean; μ_1, new population mean (Yip 2005)

The public health approach in practice

The United States of America, England, Scotland, Australia, New Zealand, Finland, and Norway are among the areas that have developed comprehensive national suicide prevention strategies incorporating the public health approach (Taylor, Kingdom, and Jenkins 1997). National strategies for suicide prevention in these areas shared a number of common elements (US Department of Health and Human Services 2001). These include:

- Using educational settings as sites of intervention;
- Promotion of research on suicide and suicide prevention;
- Attempts to change the portrayal of suicidal behaviour and mental illness in the media;
- Efforts to increase and improve the detection and treatment of depression and other mental illnesses;
- Emphasis on reducing the stigma associated with help-seeking behaviours;
- Strategies designed to improve access to services;
- Promotion of effective preventive efforts with rigorous evaluation; and
- Efforts to reduce access to suicide means.

It has been argued that national programmes in Australia, Finland, Norway, and Sweden had little or no impact on reducing suicide rates among youth and the general population (De Leo 2004). Although definitive evidence to demonstrate the implementation of a national suicide prevention policy is yet to be confirmed, the establishment of a national policy reflects a commitment by the local government to deal with the challenges. It also offers more coordinated policies and measures for the community. From the experiences of other countries, we advocate the importance of incorporating a similar public health approach in preventing suicide in the Western Pacific Region of the World Health Organization, especially in countries with a large population.

Chapter 2: Formulation and evaluation of suicide prevention programmes

Need for effective suicide prevention programmes

One of the most challenging concerns in offering suicide prevention programmes is the lack of evidence on the effectiveness of prevention programmes (Gunnell and Frankel 1994). To our best knowledge, only a few suicide prevention programmes have been rigorously studied and evaluated for their effectiveness in reducing suicide and its related risk factors (Aseltine and DeMartino 2004, De Leo, Dello Buono, and Dwyer 2002, Hawton *et al.* 2001, Knox *et al.* 2003, Rihmer, Rutz, and Pihlgren 1995, Rutz, von Knorring, and Walinder 1992, Toumbourou and Gregg 2002, Wong *et al.*, 2009). Most interventions that are assumed to prevent suicide, including some that have been widely implemented, have had no systematic evaluation or are yet to be evaluated. Aside from the problem of a lack of reliable outcome measures, the majority of the programmes also suffer from a low-base suicide rate. For instance, mortality and morbidity are often used to measure the impact of preventive measures and subsequently used to establish priorities for health resource allocation. Suicide prevention, as a result, often ranks as a relatively low priority in resource allocation.

To date, only a few programmes, over decades of suicide research, have used suicide mortality as the main outcome measure. For examples, these include the United States Air Force suicide prevention programme (Knox *et al.* 2003), the Gotland study on suicide and depression (Rihmer *et al.* 1995, Rutz, von Knorring, and Walinder 1992), the legislation restricting pack sizes of paracetamol and salicylates and its effect on self-poisoning in the United Kingdom (Hawton *et al.* 2001), and the Matsunoyama study in Japan (Kawamura *et al.* 2007) and restriction of sales of charcoal (Yip *et al.* 2010). Other suicide prevention efforts, for example, have been focused largely on young people, using levels of risk factors for suicide (i.e. adolescent delinquent behaviour and substance use) as the outcome measures. The emphasis of preventive efforts on young people may reflect public attention on the strategy of youth suicide. However, the need for prevention in other groups such as elderly and middle-aged men appears to be overlooked, not to mention the lack of rigorous evaluation in most of these programmes aimed at these people.

Policy-makers and stakeholders often do not have adequate information on what makes an effective prevention programme, let alone which programmes meet this criteria. To resolve this problem, adequate resources should be directed towards evaluating the existing suicide preventions, as well as intervention programmes, to ensure that target populations are being aided effectively. Stakeholders and funding bodies should be informed of the importance of an evidence-based programme, and include the evaluation element into their funding criteria and policies.

Key elements in formulating suicide prevention strategies

Using the United Kingdom's experience as an example, four key principles of suicide prevention strategy should include (Mehlum 2004):

Comprehensiveness

- Coordinated efforts from different sectors of the community
- Three extensive levels of interventions (universal, selective, and indicated)

Empirical evidence

- Interventions should be derived from evidence-based conceptual frameworks
- Ongoing research is necessary to support previous findings

Measurable outcomes

- Preventive measures must be specific to the needs
- Services should be practical and accessible
- Intervention should be open to monitoring

Subject to change

- Intervention must be subject to continuous evaluation
- Strategies should be changed when necessary

Another important element of a programme that must not be excluded is sustainability (Heady *et al.* 2006):

Sustainability

- Intervention programmes should be self-sustaining (if the project requires long-term presence), especially when faced with a finite funding period. The longevity of a project's achievements and effects for participants should be long-term, or at least able to be maintained

Criteria for effective interventions

In the previous section, the rationale of suicide prevention strategies using the public health approach was discussed. In order to achieve effective interventions, we propose four criteria: (1) an empirically established conceptual framework; (2) clear identification of service users; (3) carefully planned interventions; and (4) rigorous and ongoing evaluations.

Empirically established conceptual framework

- Identify the risk and protective factors to the problem
- Determine the need for intervention
- Establish the components of the service model, including identification of target individuals, evidence-based intervention, and scientific evaluation

Clear identification of target individuals

- Establish a clear definition of target individuals or behaviours
- Develop mechanisms to identify and reach out to appropriate service users
- Proactively recruit target individuals

Carefully planned intervention/preventative measures

- Formulate interventions or measures based on a solid conceptual framework derived from empirical evidence
- Timely implementation of interventions
- Programmes focused on mitigating risk factors and enhancing protective factors for specific target groups (for indicated programmes, intervention should aim at reducing imminent suicide)
- Collaboration with other gatekeepers in the community
- Continuity of care

Systematic evaluation

- Identify relevant indicators and measurable outcomes clearly
- Deliberate and continuous evaluation of programme effectiveness, with improvements in evaluation methods whenever possible
- Programmes are subject to change, based on effectiveness

Measurable outcome indicators for interventions

Suicide is a complex phenomenon, involving a complex interaction among neurological, genetic, psychological, social, cultural, and environmental risk factors (Agerbo, Sterne, and Gunnell 2007, Chen *et al.* 2006, Cheng *et al.* 2000, Mortensen *et al.* 2000, Phillips *et al.* 2002, Vijayakumar *et al.* 2005a). Interventions, which aim at reducing occurrence of these risk factors, may also contribute to the reduction of suicide incidents.

Since suicide is a low-base rate phenomenon, service providers should recognize that reduction in suicide rates should not be the only outcome indicator for the effectiveness of a preventive programme (Gunnell and Frankel 1994). Other suicide-related outcomes such as a decrease in the prevalence of depression, suicidal ideation and suicide attempt rate, improvement in suicide-related knowledge, and enhancement in protective factors should also be considered (De Leo 2002, Goldney and Fisher 2008, Goldney *et al.* 2001, Gould *et al.* 2003).

Major outcomes for interventions

- **Decrease in suicide rate**

Some preventive programmes have shown statistically significant reduction in suicide rate. Most of them are interventions in enclosed settings, such as the United States Air Force Program (Knox *et al.* 2003), community-based prevention programmes for elderly in Japan (Oyama *et al.* 2006a), and the Gotland Study (Rihmer, Rutz, and Pihlgren 1995). Recent studies using suicide rates as the outcome measure showed significant changes in the rate, which provides encouraging support for using suicide rates as the main measurable outcome target for intervention (Pirkola *et al.* 2009, Szanto *et al.* 2007). However, suicide rate in itself is not recommended to be used as the only primary indicator of measuring the effectiveness of suicide prevention. It can be considered as an ultimate goal if many of the proposed risk factors are reduced or protective factors are enhanced. Due to the very low rate in completed suicides, some alternative measures need to be constructed to measure the effectiveness of any suicide prevention programme, especially for a relatively small community.

- **Decrease in suicide attempt rate**

Suicides and suicide attempts are two overlapping populations, but are distinguished by different factors, such as gender (Beautrais 2001b). Other studies showed that suicide attempt is a strong predictor of completed suicide (Hawton *et al.* 1998, Tidemalm *et al.* 2008, Tsoh *et al.* 2005). Many programme evaluations adopted using it as the main outcome measure (Aseltine *et al.* 2007, Brown *et al.* 2005; Hegerl *et al.* 2006, Mishara, Houle, and Lavoie 2005, Vaiva *et al.* 2006, van Heeringen *et al.* 1995).

- **Decrease in suicidal ideation**

Suicide ideation is quite common in the community. The younger group tends to have a high prevalence of suicide ideation and in relation to other risk factors, such as violence, substance abuse and depression (Brunstein Klomek *et al.* 2007, Galaif *et al.* 2007, King *et al.* 2001, Liu *et al.* 2005, Yip *et al.* 2004). The prevalence of suicide ideation has been commonly used as indicators for research, as well as intervention programmes of suicide prevention (Brook *et al.* 2006, Brown *et al.* 2005, De Leo *et al.* 2005, Ramchand *et al.* 2008).

Associated outcomes for interventions

- **Increase in mental health literacy and help-seeking behaviour**

  Research shows that increased awareness about suicide and mental illnesses, together with reducing the misunderstandings, may be considered as one of the suicide prevention strategies (Goldney and Fisher 2008, Hoven *et al.* 2008). Suicide rates reflect the mental well-being of the community as a whole. For instance, mental illness, including depression, is one of the strongest risk factors of suicide (Phillips *et al.* 2007). Lack of understanding about suicide and/or stigma prevents at-risk individuals from seeking needed care, and prevents those who know at-risk individuals from recognizing symptoms and taking appropriate action. Moreover, enhancing protective factors (i.e. help-seeking) and reducing risk factors (i.e. stigma) are known to be associated with lower risks of suicidal behaviours (Knox *et al.* 2003, Li *et al.* 2004, Moskos *et al.* 2007, Owens *et al.* 2005).

- **Increase in psychosocial protective factors/decrease in risk factors**

  It is also important to emphasize the protective factors such as family support, school success, and peers affiliations (Beautrais 2000, Fergusson, Beautrais, and Horwood 2003) in preventing suicide. According to a study on the prevalence of suicidality in Hong Kong, the presence of depressive and anxiety symptoms increased the risk of past-year suicidal ideation by six times. Poor interpersonal relationships increased the risk by five times, unemployment increased about four times, where debt and financial difficulties increased the risk by 2.5 times. Meanwhile, social support and healthy lifestyle reduced the risk of past-year suicide ideation by four and five times, respectively. Reasons for living also reduced the risk by five times (Centre for Suicide Research and Prevention 2005).

- **Media reporting on suicide**
  There are sensationalized or glorified portrayals of suicide in the media, which have been associated with suicides, which are called "copycat suicides." In Switzerland, the launch of media guidelines reduced the sensational and lengthy reports of suicides in newspapers. The percentage of suicide stories on page one declined from 20% to 4%, and the proportion of stories with sensational headlines declined from 62% to 25% (Hawton and Williams 2002, Michel *et al.* 2000). In Vienna, after the introduction of media guidelines, a sharp decrease of 80% for subway suicides was reported. The overall suicide rate was reduced as well (Etzersdorfer and Sonneck 1998). It has also been demonstrated the increase in the number of suicides after the death of the celebrities in the Republic of Korea, Taiwan, China, and Hong Kong (China) (Chen *et al.* 2010, Cheng *et al.* 2007a, Cheng *et al.* 2007b, Fu and Yip 2009, Yip *et al.* 2006).

- **Availability and accessibility of lethal means**
  Reducing access to suicide means is proven to be an effective way to prevent suicide (Gunnell *et al.* 2007, Gunnell and Frankel 1994, Hawton 2002, Mann *et al.* 2005). One of the explanations is that a number of suicidal acts are impulsive (Mann 1998) and by limiting the accessibility of lethal means, a self-destructive act may be delayed or prevented. Although, substitution of suicide method may occur (Liu *et al.* 2007), a considerable number of individuals will not use another available method, where suicide can therefore be prevented (Daigle 2005, Gunnell, Middleton, and Frankel 2000). One of the examples is erecting the safety screen doors in the subway system in Hong Kong (China), where the number of deaths has dropped significantly without a substitution to the subway platform, which does not have the safety screen door (Law *et al.* 2009).

- **Outcomes for training programmes**

    Training programmes for gatekeepers have been found to effectively increase the use of mental health services and reduce suicide risk among individuals with depressive symptoms and suicide risks (Capp, Deane, and Lambert 2001, Kataoka *et al.* 2007, Simpson, Franke, and Gillett 2007). It is because suicidal behaviours may be prevented by appropriate intervention: improving staff attitudes and increasing clinical knowledge are important for suicide prevention; reducing staff anxiety and increasing confidence will assist in the interaction with suicidal individuals; training staff in early identification of suicide risk will improve detecting people's vulnerability to suicide and could subsequently lower the suicide rate; and increasing the pool of staff with skills in assessment and management of suicide risk can overall complement the role of already overstretched mental health professionals (Simpson, Winstanley, and Bertapelle 2003). General practitioners (GPs), as gatekeepers, also provide an excellent window of opportunity for suicide prevention (Rihmer, Rutz, and Pihlgren 1995). For instance, in Hong Kong (China), among the suicide deaths with known contact with a GP (about 42%), 3.9%, 18.7% and 8% of them had contact with a GP within one day, one week, and one month, respectively before the final act (Centre for Suicide Research and Prevention 2005). It has been suggested that providing training to gatekeepers, for instance, the GPs for early identification and intervention for individuals with suicide risks can be considered as one of the effective suicide prevention strategies (Luoma, Martin, and Pearson 2002, Mann *et al.* 2005).

There are a few dimensions of evaluating the efficacy of a gatekeeper training programme for suicide prevention, including objective and subjective knowledge/skills test (Simpson, Winstanley, and Bertapelle 2003); attitude and self-confidence of trainees, which are often studied as an attitude self-assessment (Simpson, Winstanley and Bertapelle 2003)/self-efficacy (Lorenz, Gregory, and Davis 2000); sustainability/behavioural changes (Sanci *et al* 2002); and users' feedback is one of the ways in assessing the performance of trainees.

Examples of evidence-based suicide prevention programmes

With decades' worth of research on the suicide problem and its solutions, a foundation for suicide prevention has been set. With effective suicide prevention programmes being implemented and evaluated across the globe (and within the region), a wealth of knowledge has been accumulated, teaching us much about the possible ways to move forward in suicide prevention. This section has been dedicated to the practices, which have proven to be effective in their respective locations and have been used as reference for the general public. Eleven types of interventions from non-Western Pacific studies and eight examples from the Western Pacific Region are selected. Each example will be summarized by the four public health approach processes (as described in Chapter 1).

Worldwide

1. Effects of legislation restricting pack sizes of paracetamol and salicylates on self-poisoning in the United Kingdom (Hawton et al. 2001)

In 1998, legislation was introduced to limit pack sizes of paracetamol and salicylates sold over-the-counter to reduce the incident of deliberate self-poisoning. The legislation specified on limiting 16 to 32 tablets per sale and adding warnings of the dangers of paracetamol on packets and leaflets.

Between 1996 and 1999, the annual number of deaths from paracetamol poisoning decreased by 21% while the number from salicylate poisoning decreased by 48%. Liver transplant rates due to paracetamol poisoning decreased by 66%. The rate of non-fatal self-poisoning with paracetamol was decreased by 11%.

This study provided evidence for the rationale of restricting means for suicide. Both the rate of self-harm and costs of hospitalization due to misuse of the drugs decreased.

> **Surveillance:** Before 1998, paracetamol was available in two forms: loose tablets and blister packs. Those who attempted suicide who took paracetamol in blister packs overdosed less than those who took from loose tablet packaging.
>
> **Risk factor identification:** Those who attempted suicide and overdosed were shown to be impulsive while the loose tablet packaging made it easy for large overdose amounts.
>
> **Prevention / intervention:** (Universal) There was legislation to limit pack sizes.

Evaluation: There is a decrease in the number of deaths from overdose, liver transplant rate and non-fatal self-poisoning rate between 1996 and 1999.

2. *Restriction of hazardous pesticides in Sri Lanka (Gunnell et al. 2007, Hawton et al. 2008)*

Suicide rates in Sri Lanka witnessed an eight-fold increase between 1950 and 1995, reaching their peak of 47 per 100 000 in 1995. Several studies have shown that self-poisoning by pesticides account for over two-thirds of all suicides. Since the late 1970s until the early 1990s, WHO Class I (extremely or highly toxic) organophosphorus (OP) pesticides were the most common poisons taken in fatal self-harm. In response to the prevalence of self-poisoning, the Registrar of Pesticides began banning WHO Class I OP pesticides, starting with methyl parathion and parathion in 1984, and others in the following years, concluding with a ban on all remaining Class I pesticides in July 1995. During this period, farmers shifted their pesticide dependence on the Class II (moderately hazardous) organochloride pesticide and endosulfan, which proved to also be highly toxic to humans. As a result, endosulfan imports were banned in December 1998.

Between 1995 and 2005, the suicide rates halved. Ecological analyses show that the declines in the suicide rates coincide with the bans between 1995 and 1998, with the bans in 1984 possibly slowing the rapid rise in the suicide rates. Other national factors of suicides, such as unemployment, alcohol misuse, divorce, overall pesticide use and the civil war did not appear to be associated with these declines, although other factors may be the causes of the fall in the suicide rates apart from pesticide regulations.

Surveillance: Self-poisoning by toxic pesticides was a common means to suicide, especially in rural areas of low-income countries, such as Sri Lanka, due to its availability and high lethality.

Risk factor identification: There was widespread availability and access to highly toxic pesticides.

Prevention / intervention: (Universal) Import controls on highly toxic pesticides (Class I OP and endosulfan) were made.

Evaluation: The suicide rate significantly declined between 1995 and 2005, in concordance with pesticide regulations.

3. *Media guidelines in Vienna, Austria (Etzersdorfer and Sonneck 1998)*

Under certain circumstances, contact with or knowledge of an individual who had recently died by suicide could precipitate suicidal behaviour in vulnerable individuals. It has been found that the portrayals of suicide in media can influence suicidality in individuals exposed to such articles by prompting 'copycat suicides,' also known as suicide contagion. It was suggested that the implementation of suicide-reporting guidelines could decrease the negative effects of suicide reporting, and even become a positive force in suicide prevention.

After the implementation of the subway system in Vienna in 1978, it became increasingly acceptable as a means to committing suicide, with the suicide rates showing a sharp increase. Between 1984 and 1987, there was extensive and dramatic media coverage on subway suicides, correlating with the subsequent rise in suicide rates in the city. This had led to the formation of a study group in the Austrian Association for Suicide Prevention (ÖVSKK), which developed media guidelines and launched a media campaign in mid 1987. Subsequently, the media reports noticeably changed and the number of subway suicides and attempts dropped more than 80% from the first half to the second half of 1987, continuing to remain at a low level ever since. The total suicide rates in Vienna also declined, indicating little to no-suicide method substitution.

Surveillance: Higher suicide rates were found after extensive and sensationalized reporting on suicides, particularly on the suicide methods.

Risk factor identification: Sensational and extensive reporting on suicide could convey suicide as acceptable and could also induce suicide contagion through imitative suicidal acts.

Prevention / intervention: (Universal) Media guidelines were developed for journalists and news editors.

Evaluation: An immediate and significant decrease in the suicide rates for both subway suicides and overall suicides in the city were observed.

4. **Gun control in the United States of America (Ludwig and Cook 2000)**

In February 1994, the Brady Handgun Violence Prevention Act established a nationwide requirement that licensed firearm dealers observe a waiting period and initiate a background check for handgun sales. Suicidal individuals may have intended to shoot themselves but changed their minds during the five-day waiting period mandated by the Brady Act.

Analysis of vital statistics data in the United States of America from 1985 to 1997 from the National Center for Health Statistics showed changes in the homicide and suicide rates for treatment and control states that were not significantly different, except for firearm suicides among persons aged 55 and above (average decrease of 0.92 per 100 000). This reduction in suicides for persons aged 55 and above was much stronger in states that had instituted both waiting periods and background checks (average decrease of 1.03 per 100 000) than in states that only changed background check requirements (average decrease of 0.17 per 100 000).

> **Surveillance:** High handgun-related suicide and homicide rates were observed due to the availability and ease of handgun purchases.
>
> **Risk factor identification:** Handgun availability allowed suicidal individuals to attempt suicide within a short period, allowing impulsivity.
>
> **Prevention / intervention:** (Universal) Legislation required a waiting period and background check for handgun purchases.
>
> **Evaluation:** Significant reductions in handgun suicides in those aged above 55 were observed. Insignificant changes for suicides in young adults and firearm homicides.

5. **United States Air Force Suicide Prevention Program (Knox et al. 2003, US 2001)**

From 1990 to 1994 the suicide rates of the United States Air Force personnel rose drastically, particularly among men aged 24 to 35. Senior officials in the United States Air Force believed that suicide "represented the end of a long road of personal suffering in which multiple indicators of vulnerability pointed to the need for help." A programme was designed to detect these indicators early and reduce the prevalence of risk factors to prevent imminent suicide.

The United States Air Force first developed the programme for active duty personnel in late 1996 as a population-oriented approach to reducing the suicide risk. Eleven initiatives were implemented, aiming at enhancing psychosocial protective factors, raising awareness, improving the identification and treatment of high-risk individuals, and increasing help-seeking.

Analysis of cohorts before (from 1990 to 1996) and after (from 1997 to 2002) the intervention showed a sustained decline in the rate of suicides and other related adverse outcomes. Suicide rates declined from 15.8 per 100 000 in 1995 to about 6 per 100 000 in 2002. There was a 33% relative risk reduction of suicide. Risk reduction for accidental death (18%), homicide (51%), severe family violence (54%), and moderate family violence (30%) were also significant.

> **Surveillance:** Stigma surrounding psychosocial or mental health problems was a major barrier deterring the United States Air Force personnel from seeking help. There was also an evident need for enhancing detection and treatment of those at any risk of suicide.
>
> **Risk factor identification:** Interplay of risk factors included poor mental health literacy, stigma, and decreased functioning, contributing to lost workdays, reduced productivity, great personal sufferings and family distress.
>
> **Prevention / intervention:** (Universal/Selective/Indicated) Eleven initiatives aiming at strengthening social support, promoting development of coping skills, and changing policies and norms to encourage effective help-seeking behaviours, and enhancing the early detection and treatment of at-risk individuals were created.
>
> **Evaluation:** There was a significant decrease in the suicide rate, suicide risk, and risk of accidental death, homicide, severe family violence, and moderate family violence between 1997 and 2002.

6. Tele-Help/Tele-Check service in Italy (De Leo, Carollo, and Dello Buono 1995, De Leo, Dello Buono, and Dwyer 2002)

It was found that most elderly had a high risk of suicide because of the high prevalence of physical and mental health problems. Tele-Help is an alarm system that the client can activate to call for help any time. Tele-Check the client is contacted about twice a week for assessment of needs or emotional support. Although elderly seldom use hotline services, the design of the service effectively made the intervention proactive and interactive. From 1988 to 1998, data were collected to determine the effects of the Tele-Help/Tele-Check service on suicide. The 18 641 service users were compared to a comparable general population group of the Veneto Region. There were significantly fewer suicide deaths (n = 6) than would be expected (n = 20.86) despite an assumed over-representation of persons at increased risk. Tele-Help/Tele-Check service appears to provide support of great interest for the prevention of suicide in the elderly, of which results can be maintained in the long-term.

> **Surveillance:** Elderly individuals had higher suicide risk due to the prevalence of physical and mental health problems, and low help-seeking levels.
>
> **Risk factor identification:** Those at highest risk were aged above 65 and disabled, socially isolated, had psychiatric disorders, poor compliance with outpatient treatment, low-income, or requested admission to a social health institution, since they presumably needed more help.
>
> **Prevention / intervention:** (Selective) Tele-Help (portable alarm device) and Tele-Check (proactive phone-calling by trained staff) were recommended.
>
> **Evaluation:** A significantly lower number of suicides were found in service users between 1988 and 1998.

7. The effectiveness of training GPs has been shown by several studies in different countries

Of the many GP-based suicide prevention programmes studied, three of them have been chosen for this section such as the Gotland study (Rutz, von Knorring, and Walinder 1992), Prevention of Suicide in Primary

Care Elderly: Collaborative Trial (PROSPECT) (Bruce *et al.* 2004), and a depression-management educational programme evaluated in Hungary (Szanto *et al.* 2007).

Depression and suicidal ideation were principle risk factors for suicide, especially in later life. Considering a large proportion of those who commit suicide has contact with a GP prior to their death, early recognition and adequate treatment of depression by GPs is found to be effective suicide prevention.

Two-day programmes given to all GPs in Gotland, Sweden in 1983 and 1984 showed that the suicide rate, inpatient care for depression, and the frequency of sick leaves for depression decreased significantly in 1985. The suicide rate and inpatient care for depression were reverted to almost the same levels in 1982 four years after the programme ceased.

PROSPECT and a five-year depression management educational programme for GPs and their nurses, with the establishment of a Depression Treatment Clinic and psychiatrist telephone consultation service in Hungary, found a significant decrease in depression and suicidal ideation/suicide rates compared to the control groups.

> **Surveillance:** Depression and suicidal ideation were principle risk factors for suicide. A large proportion of suicide cases involved with depression and suicidal ideation had recent contact with GPs, who are often not specialists in dealing with suicidality.
>
> **Risk factor identification:** Depression and suicidal ideation in GP patients were observed.
>
> **Prevention/intervention:** (Selective/Indicated) Educational programmes on the treatment of depression and suicidal ideation were provided to GPs.
>
> **Evaluation:** All three programmes saw significant improvements in depression and suicidal ideation (PROSPECT)/suicide rates (Gotland and Hungary study).

8. *Cognitive-behavioural therapy (CBT) (Brown et al. 2005, Rudd 2000, Tarrier, Taylor, and Gooding 2008)*

CBT is a psychotherapeutic approach that aims to improve problematic and dysfunctional emotions, behaviours and cognitions through an active, goal-oriented, time-limited, and systematic problem-solving procedure. Standard CBT involves patients who are being taught to identify, monitor, and ultimately challenge negative thoughts about themselves or situations and develop more adoptive and flexible thoughts. Wherever appropriate, emphasis is also placed on teaching patients to monitor and increase pleasant events in their daily lives using behavioural treatment procedures.

As an empirically supported treatment of numerous mental health illnesses, including depression (Weersing and Brent 2006, Weersing *et al.* 2006), CBT has indirect suicide prevention potential, and has been altered and evaluated specifically for suicide prevention. It has also been adopted for specific high-risk groups such as suicide attempters (Brown *et al.* 2005) showing a significantly lower reattempt rates for CBT patients, who were 50% less likely to reattempt suicide than participants in the usual care group. The severity of self-reported depression and hopelessness was significantly lower in the CBT group than the usual care group. Therefore, CBT is an effective clinical intervention option to prevent suicide in indicated suicide patients, with research showing efficacy of the treatment in all ages.

Surveillance: Depression, suicidal ideation and suicide attempts were principle risk factors for completed and attempted suicides.

Risk factor identification: (Indicated) Individuals with depression, suicidal ideation and previous suicide attempts were observed.

Prevention/intervention: (Indicated) CBT for indicated high-risk patients was noted.

Evaluation: Patients who received CBT had reduced suicidal risks and improved coping skills and high sense of hopefulness.

9. ***Dialectical behaviour therapy (DBT) (Lieb et al. 2004, Linehan 2008, Linehan** et al. **1991)***

DBT is a cognitive behavioural treatment approach with two key characteristics: behavioural, problem-solving focus with acceptance-based strategies; and emphasis on dialectical processes. "Dialectical" refers to the issues involved in treating patients with multiple disorders and the type of thought processes and behavioural styles used in the treatment strategies. It has five components: (1) capability enhancement (skills training); (2) motivational enhancement (individual behavioural treatment plans); (3) generalization (access to therapist outside clinical setting, homework, and inclusion of family in treatment); (4) structuring of the environment (programmatic emphasis on reinforcement of adaptive behaviours); and (5) capability and motivational enhancement of therapists (therapist team consultation group).

DBT, since its publication of treatment manuals in 1993, has been adopted for numerous mental disorders, including suicidal patients, depression, substance abuse, and many other suicide risk factors.

Research on DBT as a suicide prevention strategy has found that after a year of care, 23.1% of DBT patients reported suicide attempts, compared with 46.7% of recipients of alternative expert treatments. Multiple evaluations confirmed that patients completing a year of DBT experienced significantly less non-suicidal self-injury than patients awaiting care or receiving alternative treatment. DBT patients also remained in treatment longer, and had significantly higher retention rates, than patients receiving alternative treatment.

> **Surveillance:** Risk factors of suicide were not effectively treated previously by common means, leaving patients susceptible to suicide. DBT was an alternative treatment.
>
> **Risk factor identification:** Mental disorders were observed.
>
> **Prevention/intervention:** (Indicated) DBT was used for indicated high-risk patients.
>
> **Evaluation:** DBT significantly lowered suicide attempts and reduced risk factors such as self-injury and substance abuse.

10. Lithium treatment (Baldessarini et al. 2006, Tondo, Hennen, and Baldessarini 2001)

Lithium is used as mood stabilizing drug for patients with major affective disorders. Long-term lithium treatment has been associated with reduced risk of suicide and suicide attempts in patients with bipolar disorder (BPD) or other major affective disorders.

In a meta-analysis that included 22 studies (involving 5647 patients who suffered from major affective disorders, bipolar disorders, and schizo-affective disorder), suicide was 82% less frequent during lithium-treatment (Tondo, Hennen, and Baldessarini 2001). In another meta-analysis (Baldessarini *et al.* 2006), 31 studies suitable for meta-analysis, involving a total of 85 229 person-years of risk exposure, the overall risks of suicides and suicide attempts were five times less among lithium-treated subjects than among those not treated with lithium (with an average study period of 18 months). These benefits were sustained in randomized, as well as open clinical trials.

Cipriani *et al.* (2005) reported a meta-analysis in which they found a four- to five-fold superiority for lithium treatment vs. alternatives (e.g. placebo, anticonvulsants or antidepressants) with regard to suicide risk, suicide plus self-harm, or overall mortality. This suggests that lithium has a selective effect against suicidal behaviour beyond the treatment of affective disorders.

> **Surveillance:** Patients with major affective disorders, bipolar disorders, and schizo-affective disorders had very high suicide rates.
>
> **Risk factor identification:** Patients with major affective disorders, bipolar disorders, and schizo-affective disorders were found to have high levels of impulsivity and aggressiveness, which are cofactors in suicide attempts and suicide completion.
>
> **Prevention / intervention:** (Indicated) Lithium treatment (pharmacotherapy) was undertaken.
>
> **Evaluation:** Rates of completed and attempted suicides were consistently lower during the treatment of bipolar and other major affective disorder patients with lithium.

11. The benefits and risks of antidepressant in suicide prevention

Antidepressant has been considered as an effective treatment for patients with major depression and dysthymia (Simon 2002), but was criticized that might also increase suicide risk, particularly among children and adolescents. It is noted that unpublished data of randomized control trials which evaluated selective serotonin reuptake inhibitors (SSRIs) indicated "unfavourable risk-benefit profiles" among children and adolescents (aged five to 18) (Whittington *et al.* 2004). Regulatory bodies, i.e. United States Food and Drug Administration (FDA) required warnings to be issued on antidepressant products' labelling to indicate risks of suicidal thinking and behaviours in children and adolescents in 2003 and young adults aged 18 to 24 in 2007 (US Food and Drug Administration 2009). The attention was mainly focused on whether or not SSRIs would cause increased suicide risk, which could outweigh benefits when using these drugs.

A number of ecological studies attempted to show the association between the use of antidepressants and the decrease of suicide rates. For example, the relationship between the prescription volume of antidepressants and suicide rates in Japan from 1999 to 2003 was examined. An increase in newer antidepressant medication prescription was associated with a decrease in suicide rates, but not in unemployment and alcohol consumption (Nakagawa *et al.* 2007). Such inverse relationship was particularly strong among males. The findings of this study were consistent with other ecological studies, such as in the United States, (Gibbons *et al.* 2005) and Australia (Hall *et al.* 2003). However, the inverse relationship between antidepressants and suicide has yet to be established. Recent evidence suggested the decline of suicide rates did not correlate with the increase of prescription of antidepressants in the United Kingdom (Biddle *et al.* 2008, Wheeler *et al.* 2008) and the phenomena of rebounded youth suicide rates found in the United States of America and the Netherlands, which were suggested to be associated with the decrease of SSRI prescription due to warning actions (Gibbons *et al.* 2007), however, were not found in other countries (Wheeler *et al.* 2009). Given the limitation of ecological studies in establishing any causal link between antidepressants and suicides (Simon 2008), findings generated from control trials are the best levels of evidence, which can identify the risks and benefits of using antidepressant for individual patients.

A review on 372 double-blind randomized control trials found that risk of suicidality was associated with the age of subjects using antidepressants. For those younger than 25, the odd ratios for suicidal behaviour or ideation and suicidal behaviour were only 1.62 and 2.30, respectively. Odd ratios declined along with the increase of age at a rate of 2.6% per year of age for suicidal behaviour or ideation and 4.6% per year of age for suicidal behaviour only. It is evident that for those who used antidepressants, there were reduced risks of suicidality among older adults and elderly (Stone *et al.* 2009).

Despite controversial discussions on the possible suicide risks among children, adolescents and young adults, the efficacy of antidepressant is considered as clinically significant and superior to placebo in the treatment of depression (Turner and Rosenthal 2008). Yet, clinicians were suggested to prescribe antidepressants to patients with moderate or severe depression in conjunction with psychotherapy, i.e. CBT. Patients' reactions to the treatment of antidepressants should also be carefully monitored and they should be educated about its side effects (Hawton and van Heeringen 2009, National Collaborating Centre for Mental Health 2008).

> **Surveillance:** Patients with mood disorders had very high suicide rates.
>
> **Risk factor identification:** Patients with major affective disorders, and bipolar disorders were found to have strong association with suicide attempts and suicide completion.
>
> **Prevention / intervention:** (Indicated) Antidepressant treatment was used (pharmacotherapy).
>
> **Evaluation:** The efficacy of antidepressant was considered as clinically significant and superior to placebo in the treatment of depression. However, increased suicide risk was also found in children, adolescents and young adults using antidepressant.

Western Pacific Region

1. *National Youth Suicide Prevention Strategy (NYSPS) (1995-1999) and National Suicide Prevention Strategy (NSPS) (1999-2006), Australia (Commonwealth of Australia 2008, Headey, Pirkis, and Merner 2006, Headey et al. 2006)*

Both NYSPS and NSPS adopted a public health approach to reducing suicide and suicide attempts initially among young people and then extended to other age groups (Cantor, Neulinger, and De Leo 1999). NYSPS specifically allocated AU$ 31 (US$ 28.86) million to support youth-specific health and social services, including primary intervention programmes, and secondary and tertiary prevention initiatives. Although there was no programme evaluation indicating that these efforts had directly led to the reduction in suicidal behaviours and suicides among young people, there was evidence suggesting that a dramatic reduction in Australian young male (aged 20 to 34) suicide (from 40 per 100 000 [in 1997 1998] to 20 per 100 000 [in 2003]) was attributed to achievements of the NYSPS (Morrell, Page, and Taylor 2007). Another study also supported that telephone counselling services for young people, which were funded by NYSPS between 1997 and 2000, showed that there were significant decreases in suicidality and significant improvements in the mental state before and after counselling sessions. These were encouraging results suggesting positive immediate impacts (King *et al.* 2003) of telephone counselling services.

The NYSPS was then extended to NSPS and put into operation under a strategic framework titled "Living Is For Everyone (LIFE) Framework" from 1999 to 2006. A total of AU$ 10 (US$ 9.2) million annually for seven years was allocated to 22 national initiatives that were categorized into universal, selective or indicated level with emphasis on young people and Aboriginal and Torres Strait Islander people. There was an evidence supporting that the annual suicide rate (per 100 000) had decreased during the period of NSPS from 22 to 17 among males and from five to four among females between 1999 and 2004 (Robinson *et al.* 2006). Evaluation was conducted in 2006 and provided evidence and support for beginning a new phase of suicide prevention initiatives in 2007 (Commonwealth of Australia 2008).

Surveillance: Suicide rate of young males was high in Australia.

Risk factor identification: People with mental illness and have deliberate self-harm behaviours were at high suicide risks.

Prevention / intervention: All three levels were adopted, including the universal level (mental health literacy programmes and public education); and the selective and indicated levels (treatment, support and post intervention). A total of 70 projects and 156 state or territory projects were funded by the NYSPS and NSPS, respectively.

Evaluation: There was no outcome-based programme evaluation for both NYSPS and NSPS, but studies showed that significant reduction of suicide rates, particularly among males were observed during the project periods of NYSPS and NSPS.

2. *Gun control in Australia (Chapman et al. 2006, Snowdon and Harris 1992)*

Firearm suicides make up a substantial proportion of overall suicide rates in Australia, while contributing to 79% of all firearm-related deaths. Snowdon and Harris (1992) found that stricter firearm legislation significantly reduced the number of firearm suicides, even when neighbouring states where legislation was not implemented found an increase in firearm suicides.

After a firearm massacre in Tasmania in 1996, which left 35 died, the Australian governments united to implement immediate gun law reforms. These gun law reforms aimed at removing semi-automatic and pump-action shotguns and rifles from civilian possession through banning importation, possession, sale, etc. of these firearms, as well as implementing a buy-back scheme for prohibited firearms, registration/licence requirement (using various checks and mandatory training course), 28-day waiting period after the firearm purchase, and strict storage requirements.

As a result of the gun law reforms, Chapman *et al.* (2006) found that there were no mass shootings for over a decade after their implementation compared with 13 in the previous 18 years, and that the rates of total firearm deaths, firearm homicides and firearm suicides had at least doubled the existing rates of decline. Yet, a marked age-difference in method choice was observed that shifted from firearms to hanging among younger males suggesting there may be plausible substitution effect (Klieve, Barnes, and De Leo 2009).

Surveillance: The availability of a highly lethal means of suicide was a risk factor for suicide. Firearms were available and highly lethal means to suicide in Australia. It was known that the reduced availability of firearms decreases the risk, and the rate of suicide.

Risk factor identification: Widespread availability and access to firearms was observed.

Prevention/intervention: (Universal) Stricter gun legislations (e.g. banning specific firearms, firearm registration requirement, and firearm purchase waiting period) were implemented.

Evaluation: The rate for suicide deaths by firearms significantly decreased according to firearm suicide trends. Significant declines were also found for total firearm deaths, mass shootings, and firearm homicides.

3. *Barrier installation to prevent railway suicides in Hong Kong (China) (Law et al. 2009)*

In 2002, the Hong Kong Mass Transit Railway (MTR) Corporation began installing platform screen doors (PSDs) all their underground platforms (71 in total). PSDs separated the platform from the railway by means of an airtight barrier. The primary purpose of the programme was to conserve energy by keeping cool air within the underground stations, and also provided a much safer environment, preventing intentional and accidental falling onto the railway tracks.

After the installation, railway suicides in MTR stations dropped by 81.6%, from 38 persons between 1997 and 2001, to seven persons between 2003 and 2007. This trend was not found in other railway networks without PSDs. This study provided evidence for the rationale of restricting means for suicide, and gave no evidence for station substitution despite unsealed stations being fairly accessible.

Surveillance: Prior to 2002, MTR station platforms had no barriers in preventing individuals from falling in the railway tracks. Restriction of suicide means and PSDs were shown to prevent railway suicides.

Risk factor identification: Those who attempted suicide appeared to have high levels of lethal intent and tend to die by suicide close to where they live, with knowledge of the local surroundings. Psychiatric care patients had higher risks.

Prevention/intervention: (Universal) Installation of PSDs was implemented.

Evaluation: A decrease in the number of railway suicides after the installation of barriers was observed.

4. Restricting access to charcoal – a suicide means commonly used in Asian cities (Yip et al. 2010)

Many Asian cities observed a significant increase in the suicide rates during the late 1990s, and in particular, there was a dramatic increase in suicide deaths due to carbon monoxide poisoning from burning charcoal. In recent years, this method of suicide has become prevalent in Hong Kong (China) and Taiwan, China, which has led to increasing concern in neighbouring countries in Asia (Lee *et al.* 2002, Liu *et al.* 2007). People who died in this method had high suicide intents with poor help-seeking patterns (Chen, Liao, and Lee 2009) and they tended to use the same method in a suicide attempt later (Kuo *et al.* 2008). These findings suggested that this special group of people who chose to use charcoal burning could hardly be reached by clinical interventions and alternative methods should be considered in preventing this type of suicide (Chen and Yip 2008).

A study in Hong Kong (China) using quasi-experimental design has recently been conducted to examine the effectiveness of restricting access to charcoal to prevent charcoal-burning suicide and assess whether restricting access to charcoal creates a substitution effect for other suicide methods. In the intervention region, all of the charcoal packs were removed from the shelves of the participating grocery stores (n = 79) and customers were required to ask the shop assistants for charcoal. The objective was to create a barrier to access rather than to remove charcoal altogether, which would not have been acceptable to the local community.

A reduction of 66.7% ($p = 0.03$) of suicide by charcoal burning was noted within a 12-month period in the intervention region when comparing to the control region, which has the similar geographic and socio-economic profile of inhabitants. Besides, there was no significant indication that less access to charcoal forced those who wanted to attempt suicide to take their lives by other methods ($p = 0.79$).

This study suggested that "means restriction" could be effective even when it did not involve "means prohibition." It also demonstrated a reasonable approach by erecting a modest barrier that did not limit individual choice that could be an effective and broadly an applicable approach to suicide prevention.

Surveillance: Significant suicide increases in Asian cities that were related to carbon monoxide poisoning from burning charcoal were observed.

Risk factor identification: People who died in this method had high suicide intents with poor help-seeking patterns.

Prevention/intervention: (Universal) Created a barrier to have access to charcoal packs by removing them from shelves of the participating grocery stores so that customers were required to ask the shop assistants for charcoal.

Evaluation: A statistical significant decrease of suicide deaths by charcoal burning was observed during the experiment period when comparing with that of the control region; and no method substitution effect was noted.

5. *Media effect in Hong Kong (China) (Fu and Yip 2008)*

It has been shown that there is a strong connection between media portrayals of suicide and suicide rates, particularly for the reported methods. As a result, the WHO has considered improving the suicide portrayal in the media as one of its six key strategies on suicide prevention, and has issued a set of recommendations for media professionals (World Health Organization 2008). These recommendations suggest not publishing photographs or suicide notes, specific details of the method used, simple reasons for committing suicide, religious or cultural stereotypes, and perspectives that may glorify or sensationalize suicide or put blame on someone. The recommendations also suggest working closely with health authorities, using 'completed suicide' rather than 'successful suicide,' only presenting relevant data, publishing on inside pages, highlighting alternatives to suicide, providing information on helpful services and resources, and publicizing risk indicators and warning signs.

Hong Kong (China) newspapers have often been found to be non-compliant with WHO recommendations or international best practices (Au *et al.* 2004), with a remarkably high proportion of suicide articles being accompanied with pictorial presentations (87.5%), compared with places like Australia (14%) (Pirkis *et al.* 2002). To combat this non-compliance, a public seminar and press conference about media reporting on suicide was organized, with at least 10 newspapers covering the event. Manuals, containing information about suicide contagion via the media and WHO recommendations, were also disseminated for free. Three months following publication, approximately 1000 copies were given to journalists and newspaper editors, either by post or media professional associations and journalism schools.

In the analysis of five major Hong Kong (China) newspapers in Chinese, two saw significant decreases in pictorial presentations and one saw a significant increase. Two papers also had a significant decrease in stories with headlines mentioning suicide (Fu and Yip 2008).

> **Surveillance:** Media portrayal of suicide in Hong Kong (China) was non-compliant with WHO recommendations or international best practices.
>
> **Risk factor identification:** Contagion-ignorant media portrayals of suicide were observed.
>
> **Prevention/intervention:** (Universal) Media recommendations and awareness programmes were implemented.
>
> **Evaluation:** Significant decreases in pictorial presentations and inclusion of circumstances of death in headlines, in accordance with WHO recommendations, were seen.

6. *Community-based suicide prevention programme for elderly in Japan (Oyama et al. 2004)*

It is known that the elderly in Japan have disproportionately high suicide rates, accounting for 29% of Japan's suicides despite only making up 12% of the population. Numerous studies have shown depression as one of the major factors to suicide, particularly in the elderly. The Gotland study (Rutz, von Knorring, and Walinder 1992) and PROSPECT (Bruce *et al.* 2004) showed that the proper detection and treatment of depression could reduce the overall suicide rates.

Oyama *et al.* designed a programme with an evaluation using quasi-experimental design to measure the improvement of the detection and treatment of depression among the elderly, and the decrease of stigma associated with suicide and depression by providing educational programmes on the subject. Elderly residents aged 65 or above were invited to attend mental health workshops where a psychiatrist conducted the psycho-education programme in small groups and provided information regarding depression and suicide risk. Group activity programmes composing of volunteer services, indoor activities, and physical activities were carried out to aid participants in developing better interpersonal relationships.

In comparing with the pre-implementation decade, both males and females aged over 65 who lived in the intervention area had experienced a reduced risk of suicidal mortality by 73% and 76% respectively, during the 10-year implementation decade. In the two control areas, there was no significant change in the risks of either males or females. Similar community-based programmes were also conducted in other rural towns in Japan by Oyama *et al*. Significant reductions of suicide risk among the female elderly were observed, but not for the male elderly (Oyama *et al*. 2006b, Oyama *et al*. 2006c, Oyama *et al*. 2005).

> **Surveillance:** Most elderly had a high risk of committing suicide. Depression was a major factor of suicide among the elderly. Stigma, poor detection and treatment of depression hindered suicide prevention efforts.
>
> **Risk factor identification:** Elderly, particularly those suffering from depression, were identified.
>
> **Prevention/intervention:** (Selective/Indicated) Psycho-education programmes and group activities were designed for bolstering psychosocial protective factors such as help-seeking.
>
> **Evaluation:** There was a significant improvement in the risk of suicidal mortality in both males and females during the study period.

7. *Integrative suicide prevention programme for visitor charcoal-burning and suicide pacts in Hong Kong (China) (Wong et al. 2009)*

After an extensive reporting by the media on suicide by burning charcoal in a sealed room in 1998, burning charcoal suicides have become extremely popular, quickly becoming the second most common suicide means, and the most common method used in suicide pacts.

A popular location to commit suicide by burning charcoal is the holiday flats available in the Cheung Chau island. It is situated 10km off the southwest of Hong Kong island and is a popular vacation site for its residents. Between January 1998 and March 2002, a total of 37 visitors (non-Cheung Chau residents), including seven suicide pacts (15 deaths), committed suicide by burning charcoal in their holiday flats giving the island a reputation for being a suicide spot, adversely affecting the island's tourism industry.

In March 2002, a local multidisciplinary team, consisting of mental health professionals, police officers, social workers, holiday flat owners and managers, and members of the local community committee, designed a prevention programme to prevent visitor suicides and implementing it in October 2002. This involved raising awareness in the community to establish proper attitudes, knowledge and skills to identify and help those who are suicidal, encouraging help-seeking, refusing suicidal individuals access to holiday flats, and improving the referral system and support/intervention services. As a result, between October 2002 and March 2006, the number of visitor suicides dropped to five (a decrease from 8.7 per year pre-implementation to 2 per year post-implementation).

> **Surveillance:** Charcoal burning in enclosed spaces became a popular means of suicide, with Cheung Chau island being a popular location for suicide and suicide pacts.
>
> **Risk factor identification:** Individuals seeking to rent a holiday flat who show depressive symptoms were observed.
>
> **Prevention/intervention:** (Universal/Selective/Indicated) Raise awareness and improve mental health literacy, restrict access to holiday flats for at-risk individuals, and improve the detection and treatment of at-risk individuals were the initial steps.
>
> **Evaluation:** A significant reduction in visitor suicides was found between October 2002 and March 2006. There was an insignificant increase in resident suicides, and no significant changes in suicide rates were seen in comparison to the islands implying no suicide displacement.

8. *Brief intervention and contact for those who attempted suicides (Fleischmann et al. 2008)*

Those who attempted suicide are known to be at high risk of further suicide attempts and completion. Studies have shown that it is possible to reduce the suicide rate in at-risk populations by keeping regular contact with patients, e.g. Tele-Help/Tele-Check (De Leo, Carollo, and Dello Buono 1995, De Leo, Dello Buono, and Dwyer 2002).

Between January 2002 and October 2005, a randomized control trial testing the effectiveness of a brief intervention and contact (BIC) treatment for those who attempted suicide was conducted, compiling data from five separate sites in Brazil, India, Sri Lanka, the Islamic Republic of Iran, and the People's Republic of China. A significantly lower suicide rate was found among individuals receiving the BIC treatment (0.2% committing suicide by the 18-month follow-up) compared to those receiving treatment as usual (2.2% committing suicide). BIC appears to be an effective, low-cost intervention to prevent suicide in those who attempted suicides for at least the 18-month follow-up period.

> **Surveillance:** Those who attempted suicide had a high risk of suicide. Contact with at-risk patients was shown to prevent suicide. Brief sessions and follow-up visits also showed promising results in reducing other behavioural difficulties.
>
> **Risk factor identification:** Those who attempted suicides were identified.
>
> **Prevention/intervention:** (Indicated) A brief education session with follow-up sessions over 18 months (at one, two, four, seven and 11 weeks, and four, six, 12 and 18 months) was conducted.
>
> **Evaluation:** A significantly lower number of suicides were found in individuals receiving BIC than those only receiving common treatment between January 2002 and April 2004.

Chapter 3: A snapshot of suicide prevention interventions in the Western Pacific Region

As suicide has been an under-researched topic in the Region, evidence on the effectiveness of its prevention is limited. Nevertheless, in many countries, both government and nongovernment agencies have been conducting different kinds of suicide prevention initiatives, which may be quite culturally specific and applicable to the local communities. Even though many of these programmes may lack hard evidence on their effectiveness and efficacy, they are valuable experiences, which can be used as references when we consider developing suicide prevention in our own cultures or countries. The main purpose of this chapter is to give an overview on the existing or active suicide prevention programmes undertaken in the Region. Although suicide prevention in this part of the world may not be as well-developed as those in Western societies, there are some innovative programmes that remain worthy to be further developed and may be used as references for replication or modification of practices in other countries or cities. Since systematic suicide prevention programmes are often found only in a few countries or cities in the Region, it is inevitably that most of the programmes cited in this chapter are mainly from Australia, Hong Kong (China), Japan, New Zealand, Singapore, Taiwan, China, the Republic of Korea and urban China. It is because there is relatively higher readiness on suicide prevention and probably more resources are available to allow better mental health care in these countries or cities. Given less attention has been drawn to suicide in most of the Pacific island countries, systematic prevention programmes could hardly be found in these areas from available publications. Some well-known suicide prevention programmes, i.e. hotline services, are not included in this chapter simply because there is lack of published information about the evaluation on the outcomes of these services in relation to suicide and suicidal behaviours.

Chapter 3: A snapshot of suicide prevention interventions in the Western Pacific Region

This chapter offers a brief summary of 31 suicide prevention initiatives from the Western Pacific Region in the form of a table. For those interventions that have been introduced in Chapter 2 will not be included. These programmes were compiled from research journal articles on suicide prevention strategies, the six awardees from the "Acknowledgement Scheme for Good Practices of Suicide Prevention in the Asia Pacific Region" (of the 3rd Asia Pacific Regional Conference of International Association for Suicide Prevention)[1], and other noteworthy programmes that were known to the authors, but were not included in Chapter 2.

Table 2 is divided into 12 columns: suicide prevention programme, location, responsible persons and organizations, objectives (conceptual framework), level, target populations, method (intervention), evaluation, indicators of measurable outcomes, cost of implementation, main stakeholders, and main references.

The columns "Suicide prevention programme," "Location," "Responsible parties" and "Main references" are for the identification of individual programmes and for further follow-up if more information is desired. "Location" is categorised into countries / countries or cities, with the following abbreviations being used: AU (Australia), CN (People's Republic of China), HK (Hong Kong, China), JP (Japan), KR (Republic of Korea), NZ (New Zealand), SG (Singapore), TW (Taiwan, China). It is important to note that not all studies can be generalized to other countries or regions. Therefore, when considering implementing a similar intervention in a respective area, careful consideration and prior testing (e.g. a pilot programme) should be invested before a full programme is launched.

The columns "Objectives (conceptual framework)," "Target population," "Method (intervention)," and "Measurable outcomes" are the criteria described in Chapter 2 (Criteria for effective interventions and Measurable outcome indicators for interventions). The "Level" column indicates which of the three health care intervention levels they come under, as described in Chapter 1 (The public health

---

[1] International Association for Suicide Prevention (IASP) and Centre for Suicide Research and Prevention of the University of Hong Kong (organizers of the 3rd Asia Pacific Regional Conference of IASP 2008 Hong Kong) aimed to acknowledge good practices of suicide prevention in Asia Pacific Region. A total of six programmes had been selected from nominations made by National Representatives of IASP based on a set of criteria and were acknowledged during the conference on 2 November 2008. The scheme supported by Mr Peter Lee's Care for Life Association was to encourage evidence-based practices aimed at reducing suicidal behaviours with solid conceptual framework, clear identification of target populations, and intervention with measurable outcomes.

approach processes): universal (U), selective (S), indicated (I). The table is in the order according to these categories. "Cost" means the cost of implementation, which is an important consideration in many of the Western Pacific countries, as suicide prevention is under funded and can only implement the most cost-effective interventions. Three levels, such as low, medium and high, are used that indicate the level of estimated cost incurred by specific interventions targeted on suicide prevention. Knowledge of the "main stakeholders" is also significant in communities where the support from certain groups may be too difficult or impossible to obtain, making certain intervention unviable.

In reference to the two papers regarding evidence on effectiveness of suicide prevention (Beautrais *et al.* 2007, Mann *et al.* 2005), we decided to adopt four categories to indicate the level of evidence of all listed interventions in this chapter under the "Evaluation" column as: "Effective," "Promising," "Insufficient evidence," and "N/A" (not available). "Effective" indicates that the study showed positive, statistically significant resulting with valid controls. "Promising" indicates either notable positive results without enough statistical weight or control trials to fit under the "Effective" category, or mixed results requiring the improvement of the intervention (such as the intervention having significant effects on females, but not on males or the study population as a whole). The "Promising" category highlights interventions that have good conceptual frameworks and/or potential effectiveness, but are in need of more evidence and testing to be considered a fully valid option in suicide prevention. "Insufficient evidence" indicates lack of significant results or valid measures. "N/A" indicates no reported results.

Chapter 3: A snapshot of suicide prevention interventions in the Western Pacific Region

Table 2: A Snapshot of suicide prevention programmes in Western Pacific Region

Suicide prevention programme (location)	Responsible party	Objectives (conceptual framework)	Level	Target population	Method/ intervention	Measurable outcomes	Evaluation	Cost	Main stakeholders	Main references
1. Eastern District Project on Prevention of Deliberate Self-Harm (HK)	Police, housing management, social service providers, psychiatrists, physicians of emergency departments, and researchers	Community-based approach on prevention of deliberate self-harm (DSH) through a multi-agency working group to streamline referral procedures, enhance training of police in dealing with DSH, raise public awareness, foster community support and in suicide hotspots and suicide attempts	U/S/I	High-risk group, helping professionals, gatekeepers and general population	Raise awareness, train gatekeepers, improve treatment of high-risk individuals	Suicide rates, Suicide attempts	Promising	Low	Gatekeepers (local police, housing staff, healthcare workers, teachers, parents), government departments	Acknowledgement Scheme, 2008 (Centre for Suicide Research and Prevention 2009)
2. Reporting style for suicide stories (AU)	N/A	Certain aspects of media portrayal can influence suicidality in individuals exposed to suicide stories. Reporting style can be altered to decrease suicide rates.	U	Media industries and general population	Improve media portrayals of suicide	Suicide rates	Promising	Low	Media industry	(Cantor and Baume 1999, Martin and Koo 1997)

Towards Evidence-Based Suicide Prevention Programmes

Chapter 3: A snapshot of suicide prevention interventions in the Western Pacific Region

Suicide prevention programme (location)	Responsible party	Objectives (conceptual framework)	Level	Target population	Method/ intervention	Measurable outcomes	Evaluation	Cost	Main stakeholders	Main references
3. School-based prevention programme (NZ)	Government	Increase protective factors including problem-solving ability, decent contact with caring adults, and sense of connection with schools	U	Students and teachers who were at schools in NZ	Increase psychosocial protective factors, train gatekeepers	Psychosocial protective factors, knowledge/ skills, attitudes, training satisfaction	Promising	Low	Schools	(Beautrais 1998)
4. Depressed Little Prince website (www.depression.edu.hk) (HK)	Research institute	Improve mental health and well-being by promoting mental health literacy, increase help-seeking by showing pathways and promoting treatments	U	General population	Raise awareness, improve mental health literacy	Knowledge about depression, awareness on suicide risk, and attitude towards seeking help	Promising	Low	Government and nongovernment organizations (NGOs) that provide suicide counselling or hotline services	(Centre for Suicide Research and Prevention 2005)
5. Reach Out! website www.reachout.com.au (AU)	NGO	Improve mental health and well-being of young Australians by promoting mental health literacy, increase help-seeking by showing pathways, promoting treatment, and offering professional help	U	Youth, young adults, helping professionals	Raise awareness, improve mental health literacy, improve treatment of high-risk individuals	Knowledge and attitude about mental health issues	Promising	Low	N/A	Acknowledgement Scheme, 2008 (Centre for Suicide Research and Prevention 2009)

Chapter 3: A snapshot of suicide prevention interventions in the Western Pacific Region

Suicide prevention programme (location)	Responsible party	Objectives (conceptual framework)	Level	Target population	Method/ intervention	Measurable outcomes	Evaluation	Cost	Main stakeholders	Main references
6. Community-based intervention by the health promotion approach (JP)	Government	To examine whether a community-based intervention for suicide prevention emphasizing the empowerment of residents and civic participation has the effect of reducing suicide rates in rural towns	U	General population	Raise awareness, improve psychosocial protective factors	Suicide rate	Effective	Low	Healthcare services, general community, non-profit organizations	(Motohashi et al. 2007)
7. Prescription requirement for hypnotic drugs (JP)	Government	To reduce suicide rate by intoxication through making prescription compulsory for hypnotic drugs	U	General population	Restricting access to means of suicide	Suicide rate	Effective	Low	Government, pharmacists	(Yamasawa et al. 1980)
8. Mental health awareness (AU)	Government	Increase awareness and mental health literacy through campaigns to increase help-seeking	U	General population	Raise awareness, increase mental health literacy, increase help-seeking	Help-seeking behaviour, mental health literacy	Promising	Medium	Suicide prevention services	(Headey et al. 2006, Robinson et al. 2006)
9. Effectiveness of barriers at suicide jumping sites (AU)	Government	To examine the impact of barriers at known jumping sites on suicide rates	U	General population	Restricting access to means of suicide	Suicide rate	Effective	N/A	Government, property owners	(Beautrais 2001a)
10. Legislative restrictions on gun possession and control (NZ)	Government	To examine the impact of introducing more restrictive firearms legislation in NZ on suicides involving firearms	U	General population	Restricting access to suicide means	Suicide rate	Promising	Low	Government	(Beautrais, Fergusson, and Horwood 2006)

Chapter 3: A snapshot of suicide prevention interventions in the Western Pacific Region

Suicide prevention programme (location)	Responsible party	Objectives (conceptual framework)	Level	Target population	Method/ intervention	Measurable outcomes	Evaluation	Cost	Main stakeholders	Main references
11. Effectiveness of restricting prescription of hypnotic sedatives (AU)	Government	To reduce suicide rate by intoxication through restricting prescription for sedatives	U	General population	Restricting access to suicide means	Suicide rate	Effective	Low	Government, pharmacists	(Oliver and Hetzel 1972)
12. Regulations on motor vehicle exhaust gas (AU)	Government	To determine whether the suicide rate fell after lower carbon dioxide emission levels were required from certain vehicles through new exhaust regulations	U	General population	Restricting access to suicide means	Suicide rate	Promising	Medium, costs for design of the new model of vehicles	N/A	(Brennan, Routley, and Ozanne-Smith 2006)
13. The Sports Challenge international programme (AU, SG)	NGO	Groups of selected children or adolescents or the whole classes receive instruction from trained high-profile athletes or mentors. The various programmes on offer range from a 10-week, two times per hour sessions per week for selected youth, to the whole class programmes ranging from one to six weeks duration teaching psychosocial skills	U/S	Youth with social risk factors (low sense of basic trust, sense of shame, doubt, inferiority and low self-esteem)	Improve treatment of high-risk individuals, increase psychosocial protective factors	Self-esteem and self-concept scores	Promising	Low/ medium	Programme implementers, schools	(Tester, Watkins, and Rouse 1999)

Towards Evidence-Based Suicide Prevention Programmes

Chapter 3: A snapshot of suicide prevention interventions in the Western Pacific Region

Suicide prevention programme (location)	Responsible party	Objectives (conceptual framework)	Level	Target population	Method/ intervention	Measurable outcomes	Evaluation	Cost	Main stakeholders	Main references
14. The Esperance primary prevention of suicide project (AU)	Local community	Increase the ability, confidence and willingness of general practitioners and community health staff to detect and help a person at suicide risk. Decrease deliberately self-harm cases with analgesics by restricting quantity sold, improve media-related suicide factors	U/S	Gatekeepers, outlets selling over-the-counter analgesics, media industries and the general population	Training gatekeepers, restricting access to suicide means, improve media portrayal of suicide	Mental health literacy, help-seeking behaviour, media reporting, availability of lethal means	Promising	Low	Local community (service providers), pharmaceutical companies, media industry	(Slaven and Kisely 2002)
15. Taiwan Suicide Prevention Center (TSPC) (TW)	Government	Standardize the national suicide report format and care delivery system, improve mental health service quality, and organize community support networks. The Center will offer a helping hand for individuals who have attempted suicide.	U/S	General population, high-risk groups	Improve reporting format on suicide and suicide attempt, delivery of care and build community support	Suicide and suicide attempt rates	N/A	Medium	Health care providers, NGOs	(Lee et al. 2006)

Chapter 3: A snapshot of suicide prevention interventions in the Western Pacific Region

Suicide prevention programme (location)	Responsible party	Objectives (conceptual framework)	Level	Target population	Method/ intervention	Measurable outcomes	Evaluation	Cost	Main stakeholders	Main references
16. Hotline for Mental Health (HMH) in Shanghai (CN)	Health care services	HMH is a free hotline for those experiencing acute situations and interpersonal stresses, or life cycle and transitional changes. The purpose is to restore their mental equilibrium, improve their social readjustment, and teach and train their coping skills.	S	General population	Improve treatment of high-risk individuals	Caller mental state self-assessment	Promising	Low	Service operators	(Jianlin 1995)
17. Kids Help Line (KHL) (AU)	Government	KHL is a nationwide telephone counselling service for callers under 18. It operates 24 hours a day, seven days a week, from a single centre in Brisbane. Counsellors were recruited and trained to empower callers or refer them on other appropriate bodies if imminent risk is identified.	S	General population under 18	Improve treatment of high-risk individuals	Caller mental state self-assessment from beginning to end of the calls, suicidal ideation	Effective	Low/ medium	Service operator (suicide prevention services)	(King et al. 2003)

Chapter 3: A snapshot of suicide prevention interventions in the Western Pacific Region

Suicide prevention programme (location)	Responsible party	Objectives (conceptual framework)	Level	Target population	Method/ intervention	Measurable outcomes	Evaluation	Cost	Main stakeholders	Main references
18. Men and Women's Joint Intervention in Life Crisis (CN)	NGO	Promote gender equality, reduce suicide rate, increase residents' ability to deal with conflicts, and improve social support system	S	Villagers, particularly those in high-risk groups, their relatives and friends	Increase psychosocial protective factors	Suicide rates, suicide attempts	Promising	Low	Programme organizers, established local groups	Acknowledgement Scheme, 2008 (Centre for Suicide Research and Prevention 2009)
19. Parenting Adolescents: A Creative Experience (PACE) (AU)	NGO	Reduce risk factors for suicide among adolescents by empowering parents with group problem-solving skills and assisting one another to improve communication skills and relationships with adolescents	S	Parents in selected schools	Increase psychosocial protective factors	Maternal care, conflicts with parents, substance use, delinquency	Effective	Medium	Schools, parents	(Toumbourou and Gregg 2002)
20. Suicide prevention programme for adolescents (KR)	Research institute	Enhance early detection of potential-risk adolescents, help-seeking in the community, and early intervention to adolescents with potential suicide risk	S	High-risk youth group, helping professionals	Raise awareness, improve identification and treatment of high-risk individuals	Suicidal ideation, depression/ self-esteem	Promising	Medium	Suicide prevention services	Acknowledgement Scheme, 2008 (Centre for Suicide Research and Prevention 2009)

Chapter 3: A snapshot of suicide prevention interventions in the Western Pacific Region

Suicide prevention programme (location)	Responsible party	Objectives (conceptual framework)	Level	Target population	Method/ intervention	Measurable outcomes	Evaluation	Cost	Main stakeholders	Main references
21. Regional Trainers Sustainability Plan (RTSP) (AU)	Government	To raise gatekeepers' awareness and teach skills needed to identify suicidal risk, intervene appropriately and prevent suicide, aim to create self-sustaining knowledge networks across the Region	S	Practitioners who may come across people with high suicidal risk	Training gatekeepers	Self-efficacy	Insufficient evidence	N/A	Suicide prevention services	(Kaleveld and English 2005)
22. Suicide prevention in Aboriginal communities – gatekeeper training) (AU)	Research institute, local community	Concern over the high rate of suicide among aboriginal people on the south coast of New South Wales to the development of a project aimed at preventing youth suicide through gatekeeper training in the aboriginal communities of the Shoalhaven.	S	Community gatekeepers	Training gatekeepers	Mental health literacy, attitudes, and ability to identify suicidality	Promising	N/A	Aboriginal community, suicide prevention services	(Capp, Deane, and Lambert 2001)
23. Training GPs to recognize and respond to psychological distress and suicidal ideation in youth (AU)	Government	One-day training course for GPs	S	Youth (through GPs)	Training gatekeepers	Suicidality identification and patient management strategies	Promising	Low	N/A	(Pfaff, Acres, and McKelvey 2001)

Chapter 3: A snapshot of suicide prevention interventions in the Western Pacific Region

Suicide prevention programme (location)	Responsible party	Objectives (conceptual framework)	Level	Target population	Method/ intervention	Measurable outcomes	Evaluation	Cost	Main stakeholders	Main references
24. Suicide prevention education for nurses (HK)	Research institute	Education programme on nurses' knowledge, attitude and competence about suicide prevention and management for patients with suicide attempts or ideation and their families	S	Nurses	Training gatekeepers	Mental health literacy, attitudes, skills of nurses towards suicidal patients	Insufficient evidence	Low	Hospital	(Chan, Chien, and Tso 2008)
25. Suicide prevention training workshop for traumatic brain injury (TBI) staff (AU)	Healthcare services	To evaluate a suicide prevention training workshop for staff working on the TBI field and develop new measures for evaluation of similar training in the future	S	Multidisciplinary TBI rehabilitation and disability staff	Training gatekeepers	Objective knowledge test, self-assessment of knowledge or skills and attitudes	Effective	Low	Hospital	(Simpson, Winstanley, and Bertapelle 2003)
26. Qigong for depressed elderly with chronic physical illnesses (HK)	Research institute	Qigong, a form of Chinese therapeutics, is an alternative intervention to alleviate depression and improve psychosocial well-being. It is also easy to learn and is not physically demanding, making it ideal for more physically weak and cognitively impaired elderly.	S/I	Elderly with chronic physical illness	Improve treatment of high-risk mental illness	Mental state self-assessment	Promising	N/A	N/A	(Tsang, Cheung, and Lak 2002)

Chapter 3: A snapshot of suicide prevention interventions in the Western Pacific Region

Suicide prevention programme (location)	Responsible party	Objectives (conceptual framework)	Level	Target population	Method/ intervention	Measurable outcomes	Evaluation	Cost	Main stakeholders	Main references
27. Community-based psychiatric rehabilitation (CN)	Research institute	To evaluate the effectiveness of the community mental health services and their culture-specific characteristics	I	Psychiatric outpatients	Community-based rehabilitation	Objective psychosocial evaluation	Effective	N/A	N/A	(Zhang, Yan, and Phillips 1994)
28. Community psychiatric nursing services (CPNS) (HK)	Health care services	Interpersonal interventions provided by trained mental health in patient aftercare may reduce difficulties during rehabilitation such as frustration, hopelessness, and/or self-harm.	I	Psychiatric patients with the nursing care need at home or rehabilitation services	Improve treatment of high-risk individuals	N/A	N/A	Medium/ high	Health care services	(Chan et al. 2000, Ng, Chan, and MacKenzie 2000)
29. Postcards from the EDge project (AU)	Research institute	Non-obligatory intervention using eight postcards over 12 months, along with standard treatment to reduce repetitions of hospital treatment of deliberate self-poisoning.	I	Patients of deliberate self-poisoning presented to toxicology service	Improve treatment of high-risk individuals	Suicide attempts	Promising	Low	Health care services	(Carter et al. 2005)

Towards Evidence-Based Suicide Prevention Programmes

Chapter 3: A snapshot of suicide prevention interventions in the Western Pacific Region

Suicide prevention programme (location)	Responsible party	Objectives (conceptual framework)	Level	Target population	Method/ intervention	Measurable outcomes	Evaluation	Cost	Main stakeholders	Main references
30. WHO-Suicide Prevention: SUPRE-MISS in China (AU)	Healthcare services, WHO	Reduce mortality and morbidity associated with suicidal behaviours, increase awareness about the burden of suicidal behaviours, and improve efficiency of general health care services	I	Those who attempted suicide	Improve treatment of high-risk individuals	Suicide ideation, psychosocial factors	Promising	Medium/ high	Health care services/suicide prevention services	Acknowledgement Scheme, 2008 (Centre for Suicide Research and Prevention 2009)
31. LifeSPAN (AU)	Research institute	Through initial engagement, suicide risk assessment, cognitive modules, and a final closure, LifeSPAN aims to reduce suicidality inpatient. It draws on the experience at Early Psychosis Prevention and Intervention Centre (EPPIC) with cognitively oriented therapy for early psychosis (COPE) and suicide prevention manuals.	I	Acutely suicidal youth with severe mental illness	Improve treatment of high-risk mental illness	Suicide ideation, psychosocial factors	Promising	Medium/ high	Suicide prevention services	(Power et al. 2003)

Chapter 4: Priority

In the previous chapters, we discussed some of the notable suicide prevention programmes from using public health approach. We also listed the criteria for effective interventions and relevant outcome indicators that could point to the right direction of reducing suicides and suicide attempts. Experiences and opinions from different countries strongly suggest that a comprehensive and multifaceted strategy would be most likely effective in combating suicide. However, with the enormous amount of work and challenges, together with limited resources, which have been a particular concern in Western Pacific Region, it is necessary to set-up priority works so that people who are interested in suicide prevention can have a clearly defined aim and assessment criteria on areas that need swift action.

The public health approach of suicide prevention aims to prevent illness, disability, and premature death through early and active intervention. It provides a strong framework for creating an effective, concerted effort across different sectors to prevent suicide. In particular, public health approach combines four fundamental activities: (a) surveillance to identify patterns and epidemics of suicide and the different rates of suicide, (b) epidemiologic research to identify the chain of causes leading to suicide, (c) design and evaluation of inventions to interrupt this chain and prevent suicide, and (d) implementation of programmes consisting of proven intervention.

The public health approaches advocate a strong collaboration among various parties of suicide prevention in the territory, as these efforts need to be strategically coordinated to maximize their effectiveness. A clear identified role of each sector of the community, better identification of service gaps, stimulation of new and innovative modes of service, and the development of evidence-based guidelines for intervention and evaluation of programme effectiveness are undoubtedly necessary.

We propose that the following areas should be of higher priority, as they are the core elements that lead to the success of preventing suicides.

Surveillance and monitoring

In many countries, the reporting systems of suicide deaths and attempts have been inaccurate and incomplete or they have not been reported to allow timely intervention to take place. Without an accurate and viable monitoring and surveillance system for suicide, it makes any evaluation programme difficult, if not possible. Therefore, it is essential for a society to track the progress of the epidemic and give a timely alarm reporting on suicide so that assimilated information can be organized and analysed scientifically and vigorously to reflect the suicide rates of different populations and districts. It will provide timely, updated vital statistics on suicides. The Suicide Trends in At-Risk Territories (START) study initiated by the Western Pacific Regional Office of World Health Organization aims to investigate suicide and suicide attempts in the Region with standardized data collection procedures. This initiative is expected to have a better understanding of the problem and stimulate locally based prevention activities (De Leo, Milner, and Wang 2009). Besides, with adequate monitoring system in place, we will then be able to evaluate the effectiveness whether or not suicidal behaviours are reduced due to particular type of intervention.

Epidemiologic research

Epidemiologic research is needed to provide evidence for the understanding of bio-medical, socio-economical, and psychological risks and protective factors of suicidality of a society. It is also of great importance to know how suicide deaths and suicide attempts are accounted for the disease burden to the community and their impact on affected families and friends. The research will provide a comprehensive and updated list of risk and protective suicide factors and high-risk groups, which can help to identify the target groups, and select the most cost-effective interventions that are likely to reduce suicidal behaviours.

Evidence-based prevention and intervention programmes

To reduce the scope of suicidal behaviours, multilayered interventions must take place. In particular, community stakeholders have to be lobbied to make use of the resources available in the communities to contribute to suicide prevention. The prevention programmes, if implemented properly and desirable outcomes are observed from evaluation, they can serve as model programmes for replications in other geographic areas with similar population profiles. Several types of prevention and intervention programmes under levels of universal, selective and indicated are suggested as below:

Universal level

- Enhance the mental health literacy in the community. It is important to make use of available media channels to educate the high-risk groups, their gatekeepers, and the public to enhance the mental health literacy, encourage help-seeking behaviours and convey messages that suicide is preventable and mental illness is treatable. These public awareness programmes can be developed through collaboration with local media professionals. However, research showed that few of these initiatives have been empirically tested for their effectiveness or any negative effects and groups with depression and suicidal ideation might not have much improvement as expected (Goldney and Fisher 2008). Evaluations will then serve this purpose.

- Restriction of access to lethal means has been tested as one of the most effective ways of preventing suicides. After understanding the many emerging suicide means, i.e. jumping from a particular bridge, we then need to develop plans to limit the access to these means in order to delay the impulsive self-harm behaviours of vulnerable individuals. Balancing between saving lives and the inconvenience that may cause a restriction, we believe that limiting the access to some lethal suicide means is justifiable. A number of interventions that are related to the access to means have been demonstrated as the most effective in reducing suicides, including gun control, restrictions on pesticides and repackaging paracetamol and salicylates sizes, and installation of platform screen doors are good examples for our references.

Selective level

- Provide training programmes for gatekeepers is vital to strengthen the knowledge and skill levels of frontline practitioners and other professionals, i.e. health care professionals, GPs, disciplinary force, media and teaching staff, by working with people who are suicidal, and suicide survivors and victims of homicide-suicide through educational programmes. This is another most effective intervention in reducing suicides demonstrated in many studies. Also, it is important to encourage exchanges between academia and practitioners on suicide research and prevention work.

Indicated level

- In addition to advancing psychiatric and psychotherapy treatments, to ensure the continuity of care is also one of the important strategies in preventing deliberate self-harm behaviours. Many patients with suicide risks are often ambivalent to treatment, and many patients do not attend treatment programmes, experience poor drug compliances, or are eager to terminate treatment programmes prematurely. Around half of deliberate self-harm patients had deliberate self-harm or suicide attempts prior to the hospital admission. To provide them with better follow-up care is of great value, which can help increase the treatment compliance rate, as well as to reduce their re-admission rate to hospitals. The follow-up care should aim at providing a strong support network for these patients so as to enhance their psychosocial functioning after being discharged from hospitals.

Evaluation

As shown in Chapter 3, most of the suicide prevention programmes in this Region have not been rigorously evaluated using sound methodologies and controls. There are strong needs to develop detailed criteria and guidelines to evaluate the effectiveness of both innovative and existing programmes to ensure that the quality of suicide prevention works. While emphasizing the importance of evidence-based practices of suicide prevention, the effectiveness of any prevention should therefore be evaluated vigorously by measurable outcomes. An evaluation framework can provide quality assurance, ensuring and monitoring the proper implementation. Moreover, the framework can provide detailed instructions on how the outcomes stated in the strategies can be measured and achieved. To reduce suicides substantially, the community as a whole has to formulate a series of holistic and long-term plans that have been tried and tested as positively effective in other countries. Evaluation and outcome assessments are important in identifying the most cost-effective strategies to tackle this problem.

In view of the large number of suicide population in Western Pacific Region, one has to be cautious on resource allocation to ensure low-budget type of programmes can have high level of suicide reduction and suicide attempts. Screening for high-risk groups and then providing them with specialized and good quality services is vital and necessary. However, this alone is not sufficient to prevent suicides particularly when there is a great demand of services with limited resources. Besides, the screening process may induce negative labelling effects on those people with high suicide risks. Meeting the potential demands among the targeted population may become impossible.

A number of studies have found that a vast majority of people who died by suicide, ranging from half to three quarters, did not have any recent contact with mental health services prior to their deaths (Andersen *et al.* 2000, Appleby *et al.* 1999, Law and Yip 2008, Centre for Suicide Prevention 2009, Miller and Druss 2001, Pirkis and Burgess 1998, Vassilas and Morgan 1993, 1997). Therefore, the public health approach can help to form a more comprehensive and effective suicide prevention strategy in dealing with those with or without ever coming in contact with the mental health services. In countries or cities where resources are limited, attention should be specially drawn to developing interventions from the universal level, i.e. limiting access to suicide means, which reduce general risk more than interventions that only target high-risk individuals.

The basic principal of suicide prevention is to prevent rather than cure. These are reasons it is crucial to stop people from reaching the edge of a cliff rather than trying to save them when they are standing on the edge. On the same token, drug clot busters might be useful in providing temporary relief for those who suffer from cardiovascular diseases, but this is not as cost-efficient or cost-effective as a healthy diet and routine exercise for the whole population.

Suicide is a complex and multifaceted problem, which often involves many interdisciplinary efforts to prevent rather than to eliminate it. That is why a public health framework towards suicide prevention with participation from a wide range of disciplines, in addition to the health care professionals, should be adopted and actively pursued in the Western Pacific Region and other places around the world.

References

Agerbo E., Sterne J.A., Gunnell D.J. Combining individual and ecological data to determine compositional and contextual socio-economic risk factors for suicide. *Social Science and Medicine*, 2007, 64(2):451-461.

Andersen U.A. *et al.* Contacts to the health care system prior to suicide: a comprehensive analysis using registers for general and psychiatric hospital admissions, contacts to general practitioners and practising specialists and drug prescriptions. *Acta Psychiatrica Scandinavica*, 2000, 102(2):126-134.

Appleby L. *et al.* Suicide within 12 months of contact with mental health services: national clinical survey. *British Medical Journal*, 1999, 318(7193):1235-1239.

Aseltine R.H., Jr., DeMartino R. An outcome evaluation of the SOS suicide prevention program. *American Journal of Public Health*, 2004, 94(3):446-451.

Aseltine R.H., Jr. *et al.* Evaluating the SOS suicide prevention program: a replication and extension. *BMC Public Health*, 2007, 7:161.

Au J.S. *et al.* Newspaper reporting of suicide cases in Hong Kong. *Crisis,* 2004, 25(4): 161-168.

Baldessarini R.J. *et al.* Decreased risk of suicides and attempts during long-term lithium treatment: a meta-analytic review. *Bipolar Disorder*, 2006, 8(5 pt 2):625-639.

Beautrais A. *et al.* Effective strategies for suicide prevention in New Zealand: a review of the evidence. *New Zealand Medical Journal,* 2007, 120(1251): U2459.

Beautrais A.L. *A review of evidence: In our hands - The New Zealand youth suicide prevention strategy*. Wellington, New Zealand, Ministry of Health, 1998.

Beautrais A.L. Risk factors for suicide and attempted suicide among young people. *Australian and New Zealand Journal of Psychiatry,* 2000, 34(3):420-436.

Beautrais A.L. Effectiveness of barriers at suicide jumping sites: a case study. *Australian and New Zealand Journal of Psychiatry,* 2001a, 35(5):557-562.

Beautrais A.L. Suicides and serious suicide attempts: two populations or one? *Psychological Medicine,* 2001b, 31(5):837-845.

Beautrais A.L. Suicide in Asia. *Crisis,* 2006, 27(2):55-57.

Beautrais A.L., Fergusson D.M., Horwood L.J. Firearms legislation and reductions in firearm-related suicide deaths in New Zealand. *Australian and New Zealand Journal of Psychiatry*, 2006, 40(3):253-259.

Biddle L. et al. Suicide rates in young men in England and Wales in the 21st century: time trend study. *British Medical Journal*, 2008, 336(7643):539-542.

Brennan C., Routley V., Ozanne-Smith J. Motor vehicle exhaust gas suicide in Victoria, Australia 1998-2002. *Crisis,* 2006, 27(3):119-124.

Brook R. et al. Mental health care for adults with suicide ideation. *General Hospital Psychiatry*, 2006, 28(4):271-277.

Brown G.K. et al. Cognitive therapy for the prevention of suicide attempts: a randomized controlled trial. *Jama,* 2005, 294(5):563-570.

Bruce M.L. et al. Reducing suicidal ideation and depressive symptoms in depressed older primary care patients: a randomized controlled trial. *Jama,* 2004, 291(9):1081-1091.

Brunstein Klomek A. et al. Bullying, depression, and suicidality in adolescents. *Journal of the American Academy of Child and Adolescent Psychiatry*, 2007, 46(1):40-49.

Cantor C.H., Baume P.J. Suicide prevention: a public health approach. *Australian and New Zealand Journal of Mental Health Nursing,* 1999, 8(2):45-50.

References

Cantor C.H., Neulinger K., De Leo D. Australian suicide trends 1964-1997: youth and beyond? *Medical Journal of Australia*, 1999, 171(3):137-141.

Capp K., Deane F.P., Lambert G. Suicide prevention in aboriginal communities: application of community gatekeeper training. *Australian and New Zealand Journal of Public Health*, 2001, 25(4):315-321.

Carter G.L. *et al.* Postcards from the EDge project: randomised controlled trial of an intervention using postcards to reduce repetition of hospital treated deliberate self poisoning. *British Medical Journal*, 2005, 331(7520):805.

Cavanagh J.T. *et al.* Psychological autopsy studies of suicide: a systematic review. *Psychological Medicine,* 2003, 33(3):395-405.

Centre for Suicide Prevention. *National confidential inquiry into suicide and homicide by people with mental illness. Annual Report: England and Wales, July 2009.* The University of Manchester, 2009.

Centre for Suicide Research and Prevention. *Research findings into suicide and its prevention - final report 2005 July (report).* Hong Kong SAR: The Univeristy of Hong Kong, 2005.

Centre for Suicide Research and Prevention. Cherishing life. nourishing hope. *CSRP Newsletter*, February 2009.

Chan K.P. *et al.* Charcoal-burning suicide in post-transition Hong Kong. *British Journal of Psychiatry*, 2005;186:67-73.

Chan S. *et al.* An evaluation of the implementation of case management in the community psychiatric nursing service. *Journal of Advance Nursing*, 2000, 31(1):144-156.

Chan S.W., Chien W.T., Tso S. The qualitative evaluation of a suicide prevention and management programme by general nurses. *Journal of Clinical Nursing*, 2008, 17(21):2884-2894.

Chapman S. *et al.* Australia's 1996 gun law reforms: faster falls in firearm deaths, firearm suicides, and a decade without mass shootings. Injury Prevention:

Journal of the International Society for Child and Adolescent Injury Prevention, 2006, 12(6):365-372.

Chen E.Y. *et al.* Suicide in Hong Kong: a case-control psychological autopsy study. *Psychological Medicine,* 2006, 36(6):815-825.

Chen Y.Y., Liao S.C., Lee M.B. Health care use by victims of charcoal-burning suicide in Taiwan. *Psychiatric Services,* 2009, 60(1):126.

Chen Y.Y. *et al.* Effect of media reporting of the suicide of a singer in Taiwan: the case of Ivy Li. *Social Psychiatry and Psychiatric Epidemiology,* 2010, 45(3):363-369.

Chen Y.Y., Yip P.S. Rethinking suicide prevention in Asian countries. *Lancet,* 2008, 372(9650):1629-1630.

Cheng A.T. *et al.* Psychosocial and psychiatric risk factors for suicide: case-control psychological autopsy study. *British Journal of Psychiatry*, 2000, 177:360-365.

Cheng A.T. *et al.* The influence of media coverage of a celebrity suicide on subsequent suicide attempts. *Journal of Clinical Psychiatry*, 2007a, 68(6):862-866.

Cheng A.T.*et al*. The influence of media reporting of the suicide of a celebrity on suicide rates: a population-based study. *International Journal of Epidemiology*, 2007b, 36(6):1229-1234.

Cipriani A. *et al.* Lithium in the prevention of suicidal behavior and all-cause mortality in patients with mood disorders: a systematic review of randomized trials. *American Journal of Psychiatry*, 2005, 162(10):1805-1819.

Claassen C. *et al.* Telephone-based assessments to minimize missing data in longitudinal depression trials: a project IMPACTS study report. *Contemporary Clinical Trials*, 2009, 30(1):13-19.

Commonwealth of Australia. *LiFE: A framework for prevention of suicide in Australia.* Department of Health and Ageing. Canberra, 2008.

Daigle M.S. Suicide prevention through means restriction: assessing the risk of substitution. A critical review and synthesis. *Accident Analysis and Prevention*, 2005, 37(4):625-632.

De Leo D. Struggling against suicide: the need for an integrative approach. *Crisis*, 2002, 23(1): 23-31.

De Leo D. Suicide prevention is far more than a psychiatric business. *World Psychiatry*, 2004, 3(3):155 156.

De Leo D., Carollo G., Dello Buono M. Lower suicide rates associated with a Tele-Help/Tele-Check service for the elderly at home. *American Journal of Psychiatry*, 1995, 152(4):632-634.

De Leo D. *et al.* Lifetime risk of suicide ideation and attempts in an Australian community: prevalence, suicidal process, and help-seeking behaviour. *Journal of Affective Disorders*, 2005, 86(2-3):215-224.

De Leo D., Dello Buono M., Dwyer J. Suicide among the elderly: the long-term impact of a telephone support and assessment intervention in northern Italy. *British Journal of Psychiatry*, 2002, 181:226-229.

De Leo D., Milner A., Wang X. Suicidal behavior in the Western Pacific Region: characteristics and trends. *Suicide Life-Threatening Behavior*, 2009, 39(1):72-81.

Dorwart R.A., Ostacher M.J. A community psychiatry approach to preventing suicide. In: D. G. Jacobs ed. *The Harvard Medical School guide to suicide assessment and intervention*. San Francisco, California: United States, Jossey-Bass/Pfeiffer, 1998: 52-71.

Etzersdorfer E., Sonneck, G. Preventing suicide by influencing mass-media reporting: the Viennese experience 1980-1996. *Archives of Suicide Research*, 1998, 4(1):67-74.

Fergusson D.M., Beautrais A.L., Horwood L.J. Vulnerability and resiliency to suicidal behaviours in young people. *Psychological Medicine,* 2003, 33(1):61-73.

Fleischmann A. *et al.* Effectiveness of brief intervention and contact for suicide attempters: a randomized controlled trial in five countries. *Bulletin of the World Health Organization*, 2008, 86(9):703-709.

Fu K.W., Yip P.S. Changes in reporting of suicide news after the promotion of the WHO media recommendations. *Suicide and Life-Threatening Behavior*, 2008, 38(5):631--636.

Fu K.W., Yip P.S. Estimating the risk for suicide following the suicide deaths of 3 Asian entertainment celebrities: a meta-analytic approach. *Journal of Clinical Psychiatry*, 2008, 70(6):869-878.

Galaif E.R. *et al.* Suicidality, depression, and alcohol use among adolescents: a review of empirical findings. *International Journal of Adolescent Medicine and Health*, 2007, 19(1):27-35.

Gibbons R.D. *et al.* Early evidence on the effects of regulators' suicidality warnings on SSRI prescriptions and suicide in children and adolescents. *American Journal of Psychiatry*, 2007, 164(9):1356-1363.

Gibbons R.D. *et al.* The relationship between antidepressant medication use and rate of suicide. *Archives of General Psychiatry*, 2005, 62(2):165-172.

Goldney R.D., Fisher, L.J. Have broad-based community and professional education programs influenced mental health literacy and treatment seeking of those with major depression and suicidal ideation? *Suicide and Life-Threatening Behavior*, 2008, 38(2):129-142.

Goldney R.D. *et al.* Suicidal ideation and health-related quality of life in the community. *Medical Journal of Australia*, 2001, 175(10):546-549.

Gould M.S. *et al.* Youth suicide risk and preventive interventions: a review of the past 10 years. *Journal of the American Academy of Child and Adolescent Psychiatry*, 2003, 42(4):386-405.

Gunnell D. *et al.* The impact of pesticide regulations on suicide in Sri Lanka. *International Journal of Epidemiology*, 2007, 36(6):1235-1242.

Gunnell D., Frankel S. Prevention of suicide: aspirations and evidence. *British Medical Journal*, 1994, 308(6938):1227-1233.

Gunnell D., Middleton N., Frankel S. Method availability and the prevention of suicide: a re-analysis of secular trends in England and Wales 1950-1975. *Social Psychiatry and Psychiatric Epidemiology*, 2000, 35(10):437-443.

Hall W.D. *et al.* Association between antidepressant prescribing and suicide in Australia, 1991-2000: trend analysis. *British Medical Journal*, 2003, 326(7397):1008.

Hammond W.R. Suicide prevention: broadening the field toward a public health approach. *Suicide and Life-Threatening Behavior*, 2001, 32(Supplement 1):1-2.

Hawton K. United Kingdom legislation on pack sizes of analgesics: background, rationale, and effects on suicide and deliberate self-harm. *Suicide and Life-Threatening Behavior*, 2002, 32(3):223-229.

Hawton K. *et al.* Relation between attempted suicide and suicide rates among young people in Europe. *Journal of Epidemiology and Community Health*, 1998, 52(3):191-194.

Hawton K. *et al. Prevention of self-poisoning with peticides: evaluation of acceptability and use of lockable storage devices in Sri Lanka*. Centre for Suicide Research, University of Oxford Department of Psychiatry, UK & Sri Lanka Sumithrayo Rural Programme, Sri Lanka, 2008.

Hawton K. *et al.* Effects of legislation restricting pack sizes of paracetamol and salicylate on self poisoning in the United Kingdom: before and after study. *British Medical Journal*, 2001, 322(7296):1203-1207.

Hawton K., van Heeringen K. Suicide. *Lancet*, 2009, 373(9672):1372-1381.

Hawton K., Williams K. Influences of the media on suicide. *British Medical Journal*, 2002, 325(7377):1374-1375.

Headey A., Pirkis J., Merner B. *The learnings from suicide prevention initiatives' project: program evaluation unit*. The University of Melbourne, 2006.

Headey A. *et al*. A review of 156 local projects funded under Australia's national suicide prevention strategy: overiew and lessons learned. *Australian e-Journal for the Advancement of Mental Health*, 2006, 5(3).

Hegerl U. *et al*. The alliance against depression: two-year evaluation of a community-based intervention to reduce suicidality. *Psychological Medicine,* 2006, 36(9), 1225-1233.

Hendin H. *et al*. eds. Epidemiology of suicide in Asia. Geneva, Switzerland: *World Health Organization,* 2008.

Hoven C.W. *et al*. Worldwide child and adolescent mental health begins with awareness: a preliminary assessment in nine countries. *International Review of Psychiatry*, 2008, 20(3):261-270.

Hoven C.W. *et al*. Awareness in nine countries: a public health approach to suicide prevention. *Legal Medicine*, 2009, 11(Supplement 1):S13-S17.

Jianlin J. Hotline for mental health in Shanghai, China. *Crisis,* 1995, 16(3): 116-120.

Kaleveld L., English B. Evaluating a suicide prevention program: a question of impact. *Health Promotion Journal of Australia*, 2005, 16(2):129-133.

Kataoka S. *et al*. Who gets care? Mental health service use following a school-based suicide prevention program. *Journal of the American Academy of Child and Adolescent Psychiatry*, 2007, 46(10):1341-1348.

Kawamura T. *et al*. Survival rate and causes of mortality in the elderly with depression: a 15-year prospective study of a Japanese community sample, the Matsunoyama-Niigata suicide prevention project. *Journal of Investigative Medicine*, 2007, 55(3):106-114.

King R. *et al*. Telephone counselling for adolescent suicide prevention: changes in suicidality and mental state from beginning to end of a counselling session. *Suicide and Life-Threatening Behavior*, 2003, 33(4):400-411.

King R.A. *et al.* Psychosocial and risk behavior correlates of youth suicide attempts and suicidal ideation. *Journal of the American Academy of Child and Adolescent Psychiatry*, 2001, 40(7):837-846.

Klieve H., Barnes M., De Leo D. Controlling firearms use in Australia: has the 1996 gun law reform produced the decrease in rates of suicide with this method? *Social Psychiatry and Psychiatric Epidemiology*, 2009, 44(4):285-292.

Knox K.L., Conwell Y., Caine E.D. If suicide is a public health problem, what are we doing to prevent it? *American Journal of Public Health*, 2004, 94(1):37-45.

Knox K.L. *et al.* Risk of suicide and related adverse outcomes after exposure to a suicide prevention programme in the US Air Force: cohort study. *British Medical Journal*, 2003, 327(7428):1376.

Kuo C.J. *et al.* Suicide by charcoal burning in Taiwan: implications for means substitution by a case-linkage study. *Social Psychiatry and Psychiatric Epidemiology*, 2008, 43(4):286-290.

Law C.K. *et al.* Evaluating the effectiveness of barrier installation for preventing railway suicides in Hong Kong. *Journal of Affective Disorders*, 2009, 114(1-3):254-262.

Law Y.W., Yip P.S.F. *Suicide beyond the reach of mental health services.* Paper presented at the 3rd Asia Pacific Regional Conference of International Association for Suicide Prevention.

Lee D.T. *et al.* Burning charcoal: a novel and contagious method of suicide in Asia. *Archives of General Psychiatry*, 2002, 59(3):293-294.

Lee H.C. *et al.* Contact of mental and nonmental health care providers prior to suicide in Taiwan: a population-based study. *Canadian Journal of Psychiatry*, 2008, 53(6):377-383.

Lee M.B. *et al.* The strategy and prospects of suicide prevention in Taiwan. *Hu Li Za Zhi (Journal of Nursing)*, 2006, 53(6):5-13.

Lewis G., Hawton K., Jones P. Strategies for preventing suicide. *British Journal of Psychiatry*, 1997, 171:351-354.

Li X.Y. *et al.* Current attitudes and knowledge about suicide in community members: a qualitative study. *Zhonghua Liu Xing Bing Xue Za Zhi*, 2004, 25(4):296-301.

Lieb K. *et al.* Borderline personality disorder. *Lancet,* 2004, 364(9432):453-461.

Linehan M.M. Suicide intervention research: a field in desperate need of development. *Suicide and Life-Threatening Behavior,* 2008, 38(5):483-485.

Linehan M.M. *et al.* Cognitive-behavioral treatment of chronically parasuicidal borderline patients. *Archives of General Psychiatry*, 1991, 48(12):1060-1064.

Liu K.Y. *et al.* Charcoal burning suicides in Hong Kong and urban Taiwan: an illustration of the impact of a novel suicide method on overall regional rates. *Journal of Epidemiology and Community Health,* 2007, 61(3):248-253.

Liu X. *et al.* Suicidality and correlates among rural adolescents of China. *Journal of Adolescent Health*, 2005, 37(6):443-451.

Lorenz R., Gregory R.P., Davis D.L. Utility of a brief self-efficacy scale in clinical training program evaluation. *Evaluation and the Health Professions,* 2000, 23(2):182-193.

Ludwig J., Cook P. J. Homicide and suicide rates associated with implementation of the Brady Handgun Violence Prevention Act. *Jama,* 2000, 284(5):585-591.

Luoma J.B., Martin C.E., Pearson J.L. Contact with mental health and primary care providers before suicide: a review of the evidence. *American Journal of Psychiatry*, 2002, 159(6):909-916.

Mann J.J. The neurobiology of suicide. Nature Medicine, 1998, 4(1):25-30.

Mann J.J. *et al.* Suicide prevention strategies: a systematic review. *Jama,* 2005, 294(16):2064-2074.

Martin G., Koo L. Celebrity suicide: did the death of Kurt Cobain influence young suicides in Australia? [10.1023/A:1009629219195]. *Archives of Suicide Research*, 1997, 3(3):187-198.

Mehlum L. A suicide prevention strategy for England. *Crisis,* 2004, 25(2):69-73.

Mercy J.A., Rosenberg M.L. Building a foundation for suicide prevention: the contributions of Jack C. Smith. *American Journal of Preventive Medicine*, 2000, 19(Supplement 1):26-30.

Michel K. *et al.* An exercise in improving suicide reporting in print media. *Crisis,* 2000, 21(2):71-79.

Miller C.L., Druss B. Datapoints: suicide and access to care. *Psychiatric Services,* 2001, 52(12):1566.

Mishara B.L., Houle J., Lavoie B. Comparison of the effects of four suicide prevention programs for family and friends of high-risk suicidal men who do not seek help themselves. *Suicide and Life-Threatening Behavior,* 2005, 35(3):329-342.

Morrell S., Page A.N., Taylor R.J. The decline in Australian young male suicide. *Social Science and Medicine*, 2007, 64(3):747-754.

Mortensen P.B. *et al.* Psychiatric illness and risk factors for suicide in Denmark. *Lancet,* 2000, 355(9197):9-12.

Moskos M.A. *et al.* Utah youth suicide study: barriers to mental health treatment for adolescents. *Suicide and Life-Threatening Behavior,* 2007, 37(2):179-186.

Motohashi Y. *et al.* A decrease in suicide rates in Japanese rural towns after community-based intervention by the health promotion approach. *Suicide and Life-Threatening Behavior,* 2007, 37(5):593-599.

Nakagawa A. *et al.* Association of suicide and antidepressant prescription rates in Japan, 1999-2003. *Journal of Clinical Psychiatry*, 2007, 68(6):908-916.

National Collaborating Centre for Mental Health. *Management of depression in primary and secondary care (full guideline). Clinical Guideline 23.* London: National Institute for Clinical Excellence, 2008.

Ng D.T., Chan S.W., MacKenzie A. Case management in the community psychiatric nursing service in Hong Kong: describing the process. *Perspectives in Psychiatric Care,* 2000, 36(2):59-66.

Oliver R.G., Hetzel B.S. Rise and fall of suicide rates in Australia: relation to sedative availability. *Medical Journal of Australia*, 1972, 2(17):919-923.

Owens C. *et al.* A qualitative study of help seeking and primary care consultation prior to suicide. *British Journal of General Practice,* 2005, 55(516):503-509.

Oyama H. *et al.* Outcomes of community-based screening for depression and suicide prevention among Japanese elders. *Gerontologist,* 2006a, 46(6):821-826.

Oyama H. *et al.* Preventing elderly suicide through primary care by community-based screening for depression in rural Japan. *Crisis,* 2006b, 27(2):58-65.

Oyama H. *et al.* Local community intervention through depression screening and group activity for elderly suicide prevention. *Psychiatry Clinical and Neurosciences,* 2006c, 60(1):110-114.

Oyama H. *et al.* Community-based prevention for suicide in elderly by depression screening and follow-up. *Community Mental Health Journal,* 2004, 40(3):249 263.

Oyama H. *et al.* Community-based suicide prevention through group activity for the elderly successfully reduced the high suicide rate for females. *Psychiatry and Clinical Neurosciences*, 2005, 59(3):337-344.

Pfaff J.J., Acres J.G., McKelvey R.S. Training general practitioners to recognise and respond to psychological distress and suicidal ideation in young people. *Medical Journal of Australia*, 2001, 174(5):222-226.

Phillips M.R., Li X., Zhang Y. Suicide rates in China, 1995-1999. *Lancet,* 2002, 359(9309):835-840.

Phillips M.R., Liu H., Zhang Y. Suicide and social change in China. *Culture, Medicine and Psychiatry*, 1999, 23(1):25-50.

Phillips M.R. *et al.* Assessing depressive symptoms in persons who die of suicide in mainland China. *Journal of Affective Disorders*, 2007, 98(1-2):73-82.

Phillips M.R. *et al.* Risk factors for suicide in China: a national case-control psychological autopsy study. *Lancet,* 2002, 360(9347):1728-1736.

Pirkis J., Burgess P. Suicide and recency of health care contacts. A systematic review. *British Journal of Psychiatry*, 1998, 173:462-474.

Pirkis J. *et al.* Reporting of suicide in the Australian media. *Australian and New Zealand Journal of Psychiatry,* 2002, 36(2):190-197.

Pirkola S. *et al.* Community mental-health services and suicide rate in Finland: a nationwide small-area analysis. *Lancet,* 2009, 373(9658):147-153.

Potter L.B., Powell K.E., Kachur S.P. Suicide prevention from a public health perspective. *Suicide and Life-Threatening Behavior,* 25(1):82-91.

Potter L.B., Rosenberg M.L., Hammond W.R. Suicide in youth: a public health framework. *Journal of the American Academy of Child and Adolescent Psychiatry*, 1998, 37(5):484-487.

Power P. J. *et al.* Suicide prevention in first episode psychosis: the development of a randomised controlled trial of cognitive therapy for acutely suicidal patients with early psychosis. *Australian and New Zealand Journal of Psychiatry,* 2003, 37(4):414-420.

Ramchand R. *et al.* A prospective investigation of suicide ideation, attempts, and use of mental health service among adolescents in substance abuse treatment. *Psychology of Addictive Behaviors*, 2008, 22(4):524-532.

Rihmer Z., Rutz W., Pihlgren H. Depression and suicide on Gotland. An intensive study of all suicides before and after a depression-training programme for general practitioners. *Journal of Affective Disorders*, 1995, 35(4):147-152.

Robinson J. *et al.* Australia's National Suicide Prevention Strategy: the next chapter. *Australian Health Review*, 2006, 30(3):271-276.

Rose G. *The strategy of preventive medicine.* Oxford, England: Oxford University Press, 1992.

Rudd M.D. The suicidal mode: a cognitive-behavioral model of suicidality. *Suicide and Life-Threatening Behavior,* 2000, 30(1):18-33.

Rutz W., von Knorring L., Walinder J. Long-term effects of an educational program for general practitioners given by the Swedish Committee for the Prevention and Treatment of Depression. *Acta Psychiatrica Scandinavica*, 1992, 85(1):83-88.

Sanci L.A., *et al.* Simulations in evaluation of training: a medical example using standardized patients. *Evaluation and Program Planning*, 2002, 25:35-46.

Simon G. Antidepressants and suicide. *British Medical Journal*, 2008, 336(7643):515-516.

Simon G.E. Evidence review: efficacy and effectiveness of antidepressant treatment in primary care. *General Hospital Psychiatry*, 2002, 24(4):213-224.

Simpson G., Franke B., Gillett L. Suicide prevention training outside the mental health service system: evaluation of a state-wide program in Australia for rehabilitation and disability staff in the field of traumatic brain injury. *Crisis,* 2007, 28(1):35-43.

Simpson G., Winstanley J., Bertapelle T. Suicide prevention training after traumatic brain injury: evaluation of a staff training workshop. *Journal of Head Trauma Rehabilitation*, 2003, 18(5):445-456.

Slaven J., Kisely S. The Esperance primary prevention of suicide project. *Australian and New Zealand Journal of Psychiatry,* 2002, 36(5):617-621.

Snowdon J., Harris L. Firearms suicides in Australia. *Medical Journal of Australia*, 1992, 156(2):79-83.

Stone M. *et al.* Risk of suicidality in clinical trials of antidepressants in adults: analysis of proprietary data submitted to US Food and Drug Administration. *British Medical Journal*, 2009, 339:b2880.

Szanto K. *et al.* A suicide prevention program in a region with a very high suicide rate. *Archives of General Psychiatry*, 2007, 64(8):914-920.

Tarrier N., Taylor K., Gooding P. Cognitive-behavioral interventions to reduce suicide behavior: a systematic review and meta-analysis. *Behavior Modification*, 2008, 32(1):77-108.

Taylor S.J., Kingdom D., Jenkins R. How are nations trying to prevent suicide? An analysis of national suicide prevention strategies. *Acta Psychiatrica Scandinavica*, 1997, 95(6):457-463.

Tester G.J., Watkins G.G., Rouse I. The sports challenge international programme for identified 'at risk' children and adolescents: a Singapore study. *Asia Pacific Journal of Public Health*, 1999, 11(1):34-38.

Tidemalm D., *et al.* Risk of suicide after suicide attempt according to coexisting psychiatric disorder: Swedish cohort study with long term follow-up. *British Medical Journal*, 2008, 337:a2205.

Tondo L., Hennen J., Baldessarini R.J. Lower suicide risk with long-term lithium treatment in major affective illness: a meta-analysis. *Acta Psychiatrica Scandinavica*, 2001, 104(3):163-172.

Toumbourou J.W., Gregg M.E. Impact of an empowerment-based parent education program on the reduction of youth suicide risk factors. *Journal of Adolescent Health*, 2002, 31(3):277-285.

Tsang H.W., Cheung L., Lak D.C. Qigong as a psychosocial intervention for depressed elderly with chronic physical illnesses. *International Journal of Geriatric Psychiatry*, 2002, 17(12):1146-1154.

Tsoh J. *et al.* Attempted suicide in elderly Chinese persons: a multi-group, controlled study. *American Journal of Geriatric Psychiatry*, 2005, 13(7):562-571.

Turner E.H., Rosenthal R. Efficacy of antidepressants. *British Medical Journal*, 2008, 336(7643):516-517.

US. *The Air Force suicide prevention program*: US Air Force, 2001.

US Department of Health and Human Services. National strategy for suicide prevention: goals and objectives for action. Rockville, MD: *Public Health Service*, 2001.

US Food and Drug Administration. *Antidepressant use in children, adolescents and adults*. [6 October 2009] Available from http://www.fda.gov/Drugs/DrugSafety/InformationbyDrugClass/ucm096273.htm, 23 July 2009.

Vaiva G. *et al.* Effect of telephone contact on further suicide attempts in patients discharged from an emergency department: randomised controlled study. *British Medical Journal*, 2006, 332(7552):1241-1245.

van Heeringen K. *et al.* The management of non-compliance with referral to out-patient after-care among attempted suicide patients: a controlled intervention study. *Psychological Medicine,* 1995, 25(5):963-970.

Vassilas C.A., Morgan H.G. General practitioners' contact with victims of suicide. *British Medical Journal*, 1993, 307(6899):300-301.

Vassilas C.A., Morgan H.G. Suicide in Avon: life stress, alcohol misuse and use of services. *British Journal of Psychiatry*, 1997, 170: 453-455.

Vijayakumar L. *et al.* Suicide in developing countries (2): risk factors. *Crisis,* 2005a, 26(3):112-119.

Vijayakumar L. *et al.* Suicide in developing countries (1): frequency, distribution, and association with socioeconomic indicators. *Crisis,* 2005b, 26(3):104-111.

Weersing V.R., Brent D.A. Cognitive behavioral therapy for depression in youth. *Child and Adolescent Psychiatric Clinics of North America,* 2006, 15(4):939-957.

Weersing V.R. *et al.* Effectiveness of cognitive-behavioral therapy for adolescent depression: a benchmarking investigation. *Behavioral Therapy*, 2006, 37(1):36-48.

Wheeler B.W. *et al.* The population impact on incidence of suicide and non-fatal self-harm of regulatory action against the use of selective serotonin reuptake inhibitors in under 18s in the United Kingdom: ecological study. *British Medical Journal*, 2008, 336(7643):542-545.

Wheeler B.W. *et al.* International impacts of regulatory action to limit antidepressant prescribing on rates of suicide in young people. *Pharmacoepidemiology and Drug Safety*, 2009, 18(7):579-588.

Whittington C.J. *et al.* Selective serotonin reuptake inhibitors in childhood depression: systematic review of published versus unpublished data. *Lancet*, 2004, 363(9418):1341-1345.

Wong, P.W. *et al.* An integrative suicide prevention program for visitor charcoal burning suicide and suicide pact. *Suicide and Life-Threatening Behavior*, 2009, 39(1):82-90.

World Health Organization. *Preventing suicide: a resource for media professionals*. Geneva, 2008.

World Health Organization. Suicide prevention (SUPRE). *Mental Health,* 2010a, Retrieved 2 February 2010, from http://www.who.int/mental_health/prevention/suicide/suicideprevent/en/index.html.

World Health Organization. Suicide prevention - country reports and charts available. *Mental Health*, 2010b, Retrieved 2 February 2010, from http://www.who.int/mental_health/prevention/suicide/country_reports/en/index.html.

Yamasawa K. *et al.* A statistical study of suicides through intoxication. *Acta Medicinae Legalis et Socialis* (Liege), 1980, 30(3):187-192.

Yip. A Public Health Approach to Suicide Prevention. *Hong Kong Journal of Psychiatry,* 2005, 15:29-31.

Yip ed. S*uicide in Asia - causes and prevention.* Hong Kong, Hong Kong University Press, 2008.

Yip P.S., Liu K., Law C. Years of life lost from suicide in China, 1990-2000. *Crisis,* 2008, 29(3):131-136.

Yip P.S., Callanan C., Yuen H.P. Urban/rural and gender differentials in suicide rates: east and west. *Journal of Affective Disorders*, 2000, 57(1-3):99-106.

Yip P.S. *et al.* The effects of a celebrity suicide on suicide rates in Hong Kong. *Journal of Affective Disorders*, 2006, 93(1-3):245-252.

Yip P.S. *et al.* Suicide rates in China during a decade of rapid social changes. *Social Psychiatry and Psychiatric Epidemiology*, 2005, 40(10):792-798.

Yip P.S. *et al.* Suicidality among high school students in Hong Kong, SAR. *Suicide and Life-Threatening Behavior,* 2004, 34(3):284-297.

Yip P.S. *et al.* Restricting the means of suicide by charcoal burning. *British Journal of Psychiatry*, 2010, March 196(3):241-242.

Yip P.S.F., Lee D.T.S. *Charcoal burning suicides and strategies for Prevention. Crisis,* 2007, 28(1):21-27.

Zhang M., Yan H., Phillips M.R. Community-based psychiatric rehabilitation in Shanghai: Facilities, services, outcome, and culture-specific characteristics. *British Journal Psychiatry Supplement*, 1994, 24:70-79.